PAIN RECOVERY

FOR FAMILIES

*How to Find Balance When
Someone Else's Chronic Pain Becomes
Your Problem Too*

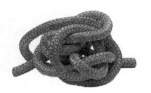

Mel Pohl, MD, FASAM

Frank J. Szabo, Jr., LADC

Daniel Shiode, Ph.D.

Robert Hunter, Ph.D.

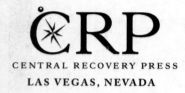

CENTRAL RECOVERY PRESS

LAS VEGAS, NEVADA

CENTRAL RECOVERY PRESS

Central Recovery Press (CRP) is committed to publishing exceptional material addressing addiction treatment, recovery, and behavioral health care, including original and quality books, audio/visual communications, and Web-based new media. Through a diverse selection of titles, it seeks to impact the behavioral health care field with a broad range of unique resources for professionals, recovering individuals, and their families. For more information, visit www.centralrecoverypress.com.

Central Recovery Press, Las Vegas, NV 89129
© 2010 by Central Recovery Press, Las Vegas, NV

ISBN-13: 978-0-9818482-3-5
ISBN-10: 0-9818482-3-0

16 15 14 13 12 11 10   1 2 3 4 5

Publisher: Central Recovery Press
             3371 N Buffalo Drive
             Las Vegas, NV 89129

Cover design and interior by Sara Streifel, Think Creative Design

To the courageous families whose
lives have been immeasurably affected
by chronic pain.

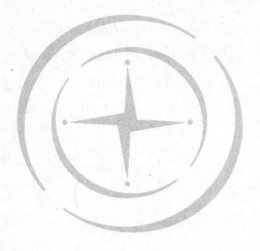

{ *contents* }

Part I Explore

Part II Discover

Part III Recover

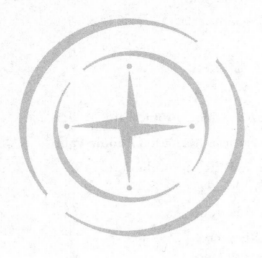

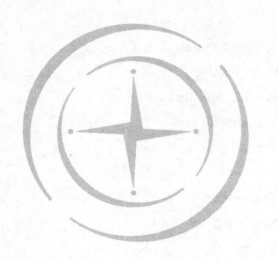

PREFACE

In 2009 we published *Pain Recovery: How to Find Balance and Reduce Suffering from Chronic Pain*, a guide written for people suffering from chronic pain who are also experiencing problematic use of pain medications. Why, then, a guide for those who live with and care about someone with chronic pain? Chronic pain is a family disease. It is impossible to isolate the person with chronic pain from the rest of the family. When a loved one is suffering from chronic pain, his or her pain becomes your pain. This does not mean you get back pain because that person has back pain; rather, it means that your overall balance in life is greatly affected and this manifests in emotional, mental, spiritual, and physical suffering. Chronic pain can be just as mystifying and damaging to family members as it is to the person in pain.

Pain Recovery assists chronic pain sufferers in finding balance in their lives, despite their experience of pain. Family participation, education, and recovery are vital to the successful outcome of long-term recovery and change for the chronic pain sufferer. Your participation is also vital to understanding chronic pain, how it has affected you, and what your long-term solution is. This book was designed to offer a parallel process of recovery for family members—to guide you on how to be okay emotionally, spiritually, physically, and mentally while in a caring relationship with someone who has chronic pain.

We stress the importance of family members practicing good self-care, no matter where your loved one with chronic pain is with his or her treatment and recovery, if the family is to stay balanced and endure the life changes brought about by the chronic pain. We hope this book will give you the tools and guidance you need to achieve this.

Mel Pohl, MD, FASAM • Frank J. Szabo, Jr., LADC
Daniel Shiode, Ph.D. • Robert Hunter, Ph.D.

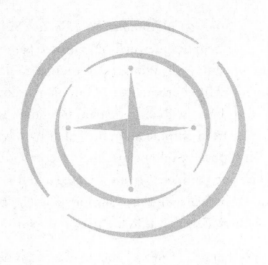

ACKNOWLEDGMENTS

We would like to express our deepest appreciation and gratitude to Stuart Smith for having faith in us and providing an opportunity for us to use our experience, strength, and hope to help others discover pain recovery. Stuart's vision, commitment, and dedication made this book possible.

To our supportive families and friends who make the work we do possible.

To the excellent editorial staff at Central Recovery Press: Nancy Schenck, Dan Mager, Daniel Kaelin, and Helen O'Reilly. And especially to Valerie Killeen, for the expert job she did editing this book.

To the skilled and dedicated clinical team and support staff at Las Vegas Recovery Center.

To Sara Streifel, Think Creative Design, for designing this book. To David Fulk for proofreading.

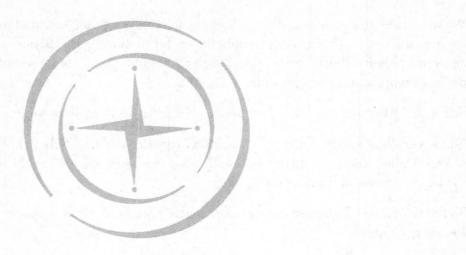

INTRODUCTION

If someone you love has chronic pain, you, too, are suffering. Chronic pain has caused imbalance in your life, and although it's not your pain, you live with it every day. Even people who are in good mental health and are well-balanced have difficulty living with someone who has chronic pain, yet there are few resources out there to help family members cope with their distress. That is why we wrote this book.

Pain Recovery for Families will show you how you can be nurturing, loving, and supportive to someone with chronic pain without losing your own identity; how to allow that person to take responsibility for his or her pain; how to be caring without being a caretaker; and how to communicate honestly even when the person in pain maintains a victim role or does not acknowledge your feelings as being equally important. This book will provide you with the principles and solutions you can practice to restore balance in your life.

Some of you may not identify with recovery because it's a term that is traditionally associated with addiction. In pain recovery, we define recovery as the process of moving from imbalance to balance. The family dealing with the disease of addiction is very similar to the family dealing with chronic pain, because both illnesses manifest in imbalances in the mind, body, emotions, and spirit. This is true for people who suffer from chronic pain and addiction as well as for people in close relationships with them (spouses or significant others, parents, children, siblings, friends, coworkers). Additionally, many people with chronic pain develop problems with use of addictive substances to manage the pain, and both conditions need to be simultaneously addressed by the person with pain and by the family.

Examples of unbalancing effects chronic pain can have on the family include:

- Loss of income/financial difficulties.
- Surgeries.
- Endless doctor appointments.
- Depression.
- Feelings of powerlessness.
- Anxiety.
- Questioning whether or not the pain is real.
- Blame or resentment.
- Increased responsibilities because of the pain person's loss of function.
- Effects of drugs the person takes for the pain.
- Feeling abandoned at functions the person cannot attend because of his or her pain.

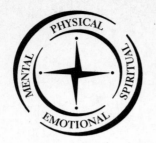

The Four Points of Balance

Pain recovery is a process grounded in balancing the person 1) physically, 2) mentally, 3) emotionally, and 4) spiritually. We use this framework to create awareness of the aspects of one's self that, when they are unbalanced, lead to problems in life. The four points of balance will help you identify the areas where imbalance has caused unmanageability in your life. These points are, of course, interconnected. To find recovery, you must pay attention to every point and the effect each has on the others. Additionally, your relationships and actions are a reflection of your internal state of balance. Developing an awareness of the points and applying the necessary corrections to bring them back into balance is where the solutions to chronic pain and other life challenges lie.

Overview

Part One includes five chapters that will provide you with a foundation of knowledge to help you develop your understanding and allow you to assess your particular situation. Chapter One presents an overview of chronic pain, and includes information about medications commonly prescribed to treat pain and problems associated with traditional pain management. Chapter Two discusses the effects of chronic pain on the family system and the pitfalls families commonly experience, such as codependency and enabling. In Chapter Three, we delve into the complex and sensitive subject of addiction. Chapter Four asks you to consider the possibility that your loved one is addicted and offers guidance on how to navigate this difficult issue. In Chapter Five, we will explain the process of pain recovery and examine the concept of balance.

Part Two includes four chapters—one devoted to each point of balance—that will help you discover the areas where imbalance is contributing to your negative experience of having a loved one with chronic pain, and teach you ways to rebalance them, thus reducing your suffering.

Part Three focuses on your recovery. Once you have identified where you are out of balance, you will be ready to take action and implement changes. Chapter Ten focuses on your relationships, emphasizing the importance of good communication and of giving and receiving support for recovery to be successful. Chapter Eleven deals with actions and gives you an opportunity to create your own action plan for each of the four points to continually bring them back into balance. Last, we have provided a focused, long-term care plan to help you proactively stay in the recovery process.

To illustrate these concepts, throughout the book we present the stories of two families' experiences with chronic pain, addiction, and recovery. You will meet Jim and Mary, married for over twenty years, and their two children, Mandi and Ross, who have all been struggling with Jim's chronic pain since he injured his back at work. You will also meet Amy and Chris, a couple who enjoyed a happy relationship for four years before Amy's diagnosis of fibromyalgia and escalating use of painkillers changed everything. We hope their stories will help to personalize the information you are learning in this book. Although your situation may be different from theirs, you will probably find that you relate to them a great deal, because the stress and difficult emotions chronic pain generates within families are similar no matter what the type of pain or the circumstances of the family.

How to Use This Book

This book is designed for you to write in, highlight, take notes on, and refer back to. It may be helpful for you to share portions of your work with a counselor, therapist, family member, close friend, sponsor, and/or other professional health care provider. Although each chapter is written to stand on its own, we suggest you start at the beginning and do not skip any chapters. Pace yourself and take breaks when you need to. If you find yourself stuck or having difficulty with an exercise, do not stop working; rather, move on to the next exercise and come back later to the one you are having difficulty with. Don't be afraid to ask for help along the way.

Now your journey of pain recovery begins, and it is time to go to work.

KEEPING A JOURNAL

We recommend that you keep a separate journal or notebook as you work toward balance. Writing can be a powerful healing tool, especially when entering any process of recovery. Taking some time each day to write about your journey can help you identify thought patterns, express feelings, maintain gratitude, and monitor progress. Documenting your experiences will allow you to reflect on successes and will help you stay encouraged and hopeful.

Part I

EXPLORE

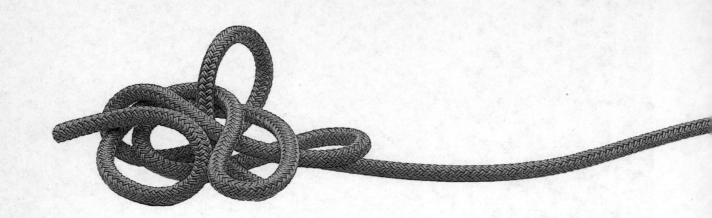

1

Understanding Chronic Pain

Jim was forty-six when he had the accident at work. He and Mary had been married for twenty-two years at that point and had deep, abiding love for one another and their two kids, Mandi, age twenty-two, and Ross, age sixteen. Jim worked as a psychologist in private practice, doing consulting for a large hospital. The accident happened when Jim was in front of the hospital. A disgruntled family member got into an altercation with an employee, and Jim tried to intercede. He was thrown to the floor, fracturing his back and rupturing two discs, they would come to learn. "Why hadn't he just minded his own darn business?" Mary would find herself asking late at night when she was unable to sleep. She would become enraged that their life had been irrevocably damaged that day, all because her gallant husband felt the need to be a hero.

Amy and Chris had been together for four years. Things had started off idyllically — they clicked immediately and had similar goals of success, romance, and eventually marriage and kids. Now, after her diagnosis of fibromyalgia, there was only a shell of their relationship. They didn't go out, have fun, or even relate to one another. They couldn't talk without fighting, it seemed. Amy felt that deep in Chris's heart, he didn't believe she really hurt like she did. He just didn't get it. Neither did her mom, her boss, or most of her friends. Chris felt powerless to help her and frustrated that she didn't seem to want to help herself. In the last nine months — since the prescriptions took hold — she was downright stoned a good part of the time. He'd be damned if he'd put up with a drug addict in his life.

These two families are confronting chronic pain, and in this book their stories will help us to illustrate the challenges of living with this widespread but underrecognized phenomenon. It is estimated that more than 70 million Americans are afflicted with chronic pain. Each person's journey is different, but some common themes run through them all. As with Jim and Amy, when a person develops chronic pain, everyone that person lives with or has a close relationship with is likely to suffer.

A range of difficult and stressful emotions often accompany the pain problem, such as fear, helplessness, frustration, anxiety, depression, grief, and anger. Lifestyle changes and prolonged stress brought on by Jim's condition are taking a heavy physical, mental, emotional, and spiritual toll on Mary, Mandi, and Ross, and causing communication to break down. Chris's attitudes toward Amy's pain and her dependence on prescription painkillers have caused a rift between them and threatened their relationship. But there are many things families can do to better cope with the unbalancing effects of chronic pain. A good starting point is to learn as much as you can about chronic pain and your family member's specific condition.

A Pain Primer

Pain is an intriguing phenomenon, the source of consternation, irritation, and suffering for millions since the beginning of time. It alerts us that something is wrong—that there is damage or threat of damage to our tissues. Pain is usually produced at the site of an injury and is processed in our complex, computerlike nervous system, causing a vast array of physical and emotional responses. The simplest response is to withdraw from the source of pain and then to protect the area that hurts.

Pain occurs in the body as a result of the interaction of nerve cells, the spinal cord, and the brain (together known as the nervous system). Interactions of a multitude of chemicals, including endorphins, prostaglandins, and neurotransmitters, with electrical impulses coming from the nerve cells create the pain experience, and also pain relief. The brain is exquisitely complex. The part of the brain that processes pain impulses, mainly the thalamus, interacts with other areas of the brain that govern memory, emotions, alertness, movement, blood pressure, hormone levels, and hundreds of other functions. The net effect, in a split second—a composite result of many inputs and outputs—is the experience of pain. Needless to say, this system is efficient beyond that of the most sophisticated computer; however, in the case of chronic pain, the system has gone awry.

There are two types of pain, acute and chronic. In acute pain, the computer functions properly, as it was meant to. With chronic pain, on the other hand, it is as if the computer has been affected by a nasty virus, turning previously healthy and necessary mechanisms into overactive and inefficient impulses that disrupt normal function. Acute pain is time-limited—usually gone within a few hours to days. It may last weeks to a few months, but it eventually goes away. Acute pain can be associated with fractured bones, sore teeth, bruises, cuts, surgeries and their aftermath, infections, and a variety of other injuries and conditions. It exists when there has been damage, and as the damage heals, the pain subsides and eventually resolves, and life returns to the way it was before. Acute pain is part of the body's "response-to-injury" system, which causes us to try to put an end to the offending, pain-causing experience. We also learn from painful experiences and are less likely to do something that causes pain (although later, as we explain addiction, you will see that this is not true in all cases).

Chronic pain continues beyond three to six months and has outlived any useful function. It should have gone away, but persists. It is the exaggerated response of the nervous system to damage, as in Jim's case, but also to other conditions and situations that occur in the brain, as Amy experiences. It is often pain out of proportion to the prior injury or damage. Sometimes a condition will develop for no apparent reason, and there is not even a clear physical basis for the protracted pain. This is not to say that the pain is in any way unreal or imagined, which was the crux of the problem for Chris, who just didn't buy that Amy's pain was real. In actuality, Amy's body simply responded differently over time to certain conditions, damage, or injury. The result is pain that won't quit.

Pain, as we experience it, is the net effect of tissue disturbance, transmission to and from the brain, and extensive processing and modifying of the pain signal. With chronic pain, the signal and its transmission are often distorted. So, despite the fact that Jim's broken back had healed and the "need" for pain (protection, withdrawal, avoiding further injury) had passed, he still was hurting.

Chronic pain is usually neuropathic, meaning associated with disturbances of the nervous system. Often the character of chronic pain differs from that of acute pain (called nociceptive pain), which is usually sharp, aching, or throbbing, and comes from sprains, fractures, burns, bruises, or other forms of tissue damage. Jim experienced a burning sensation and troublesome numbness, especially traveling into his right leg. Neuropathic pain can have a lightning-bolt sensation or an electrical quality. With neuropathic pain, people may experience allodynia, which is pain from something that normally doesn't cause pain, such as light touch or a breeze across the skin. Also associated with neuropathic pain is hyperalgesia, meaning more pain than would normally be caused by a stimulus. This kind of pain may be difficult to localize, and the source of the pain may be widespread or changing. Amy had excruciating tenderness at certain trigger points, a hallmark of fibromyalgia.

> **Chronic pain is pain that continues beyond three to six months, has outlived any useful function, and may or may not have a clear physical basis.**

Amy's pain, as with many others who experience chronic pain, was a part of a phenomenon called central pain. This is the result of poorly understood changes in the nervous system's perception of pain. With central pain, the "volume knob" for the perception of pain is turned up higher than normal. It is the increased "volume" that causes a normally light-touch sensation to be an awful sensation for Amy.

The worst news about chronic pain is that—though it may wax and wane—in most cases it doesn't go away. Chronic pain is one of the major reasons people go to doctors and is said to be the most costly health care problem in America. Countless others like Chris, Mary, Mandi, and Ross are affected by living in a household with or caring for someone with chronic pain. Obviously, if you are reading this book, your life has been affected significantly by chronic pain.

{ *exercise* }
{ 1.1 }

Who Is Your Person with Pain? _____

You are probably reading this with a specific person, perhaps more than one person, in mind. Identify the person in your life who has chronic pain and describe your relationship with him/her/them.

_____

_____

_____

_____

_____

_____

From this point on, where you see _____, write in the name of the person(s) you identified in this exercise.

{ *exercise* }
{ 1.2 }

Types of Chronic Pain _____

Here is just a partial list of the many potential causes of chronic pain. Find the cause(s) of _____'s pain and check it/them off or write them in the space provided if the causes are not listed.

_____ Back, neck, and joint pain, which can result from tension, muscle injury, nerve damage, disc disease, or arthritis.

_____ Burn pain, which can continue long after a burn wound has healed.

_____ Chronic pelvic pain, which refers to any pain in your pelvic region (the area between your belly button and your hips) from tumors, infections, or scar tissue.

_____ Cancer pain, which can result from the growth of a tumor with pressure on nerves, from treatment of the disease (chemotherapy or radiation treatments), or from other effects on the body.

_____ Infections that didn't respond to treatment, which can occur almost anywhere in the body.

_____ Chronic abdominal pain (with or without physical explanation or findings), ulcers, gallbladder disease, pancreatitis, and gastroesophageal reflux disease (GERD).

_____ Inflammatory bowel disease, irritable bowel syndrome, or other intestinal problems.

_____ Bursitis, which can affect any joint, most commonly knees, shoulders, hips, elbows, or wrists.

_____ Head and facial pain, which can be caused by dental problems, temporomandibular joint (TMJ) disorders, trigeminal neuralgia, or conditions affecting the nerves in the face.

_____ Chronic headaches, such as migraines, cluster headaches, and tension headaches.

_____ Multiple sclerosis, which can include numbness, aching, or pain.

_____ Angina or chest pain from heart disease.

_____ Uterine fibroid tumors (growths in the womb that can be associated with bleeding).

_____ Chronic obstructive pulmonary disease (COPD) or emphysema.

_____ Peripheral vascular disease (inadequate blood circulation to arms and legs).

_____ Ankylosing spondylitis (severe arthritis with restriction of spinal movement).

_____ Myofascial pain syndromes (heightened experience of pain coming from the brain, which impacts soft tissue and muscles). This includes fibromyalgia, which is characterized by tenderness in multiple trigger points, widespread muscle pain, fatigue, and stiffness.

_____ Whiplash that doesn't go away after an accident.

_____ Broken bones that healed incompletely or in the wrong position.

_____ Arthritis (rheumatoid, osteo, or other forms), which can affect any joint, including hips, knees, neck, back, fingers, wrists, and feet.

_____ Neuropathy from a variety of conditions, including HIV/AIDS, injury, and cancer.

_____ Other: _____

_____

_____

_____

ALL PAIN IS REAL

Since chronic pain frequently cannot be seen or measured, unlike a broken arm (acute pain), doctors, colleagues, friends, or family members sometimes question or doubt the sufferer's pain. Chris is a good example of this, doubting the validity of Amy's fibromyalgia pain. In order to be helpful, it is extremely important to acknowledge that *all pain is real.* The nervous system is made up of electrical circuits modified by chemical neurotransmitters, and the sum total of how these billions of cells interact is our essence—our joy, fear, sight, smell, and all sensations, as well as the experience of pain.

The Subjective Nature of Pain

For some people, like Amy and Jim, chronic pain can be disabling, while for others it is merely annoying. Jim stays in bed when he hurts; Amy pushes through the pain some days and goes about her business. Each person's unique experience of pain is based on many factors, including:

- Age.
- Ethnicity.
- Religion.
- Circumstances (context).
- Stereotypes.
- Prior experience with pain.

- Gender.
- Culture.
- Environment.
- Attitudes.
- Social influences.
- Hormone levels.

There are countless examples of how these factors can influence a person's perception of pain. For instance, studies have identified a number of gender differences regarding pain perception. Women are likely to experience pain more often and with greater intensity, while men are less likely to seek help for and express their pain (suffering in silence with a "stiff upper lip"). Attitudes toward and expressions of pain also vary among different cultures. For example, Western cultures tend to have a much lower threshold for pain than some Asian cultures, where pain is viewed as having spiritual meaning.

Prior painful experiences can also influence pain perception. Jim expected to have so much pain at a family picnic, because he had previously, that he just refused to get up and go with Mary and the kids—another serious disappointment for this damaged family. In fact, Jim would come to learn that believing that his pain would be worse based on the last time he was up and around for four hours actually created more pain for him and more suffering for his family.

And just as the experience of pain is entirely subjective for Jim, the responses of Mary and the kids (and other family, friends, coworkers) to his pain vary widely.

Pain Is Subjective

{ *exercise* 1.3 }

Describe how the personal factors listed on the previous page may have affected _____'s experience of pain. Include any factors not listed that you believe affected his or her pain.

_____

_____

_____

_____

_____

_____

_____

_____

Describe your personal issues and assumptions about pain. How do these things affect your feelings about _____'s pain?

_____

_____

_____

_____

_____

_____

Manifestations of Chronic Pain

Chronic pain can be a troublesome annoyance or a devastating curse that interrupts life functions, relationships, employment, and most things in life that bring people satisfaction. In Jim's case, it took over his life and the lives of his family, it consumed them, and it threatened Jim's well-being and the well-being of Mary, Mandi, and Ross. For Amy, traditional pain management (medication and physical interventions) did not help sufficiently. She developed a constellation of troubling symptoms.

{ *exercise* 1.4 }

Pain Manifestations _____

Here is a list of some of the manifestations of chronic pain. Please check off those you believe _____ has experienced.

____ Pain that has lasted for more than six months.

____ Feelings of depression, anger, worry, discouragement, and irritability.

____ Sleep difficulties.

____ Financial problems.

____ Problems relating to others, causing significant disturbance in relationships.

____ Inability to tolerate physical activities.

____ Withdrawal from social activities.

____ Inability to concentrate.

____ Poor memory.

____ Isolation from support systems, including family, friends, and coworkers.

____ A decrease in sexual activity or performance.

____ A decrease in self-esteem.

____ Secondary physical problems.

____ Problematic use of pain medications and/or alcohol or addiction.

____ Avoiding work and leisure activities.

____ Negative attitudes concerning everyday life.

____ Other: _____

_____

Write about the feelings that come up as you review this list.

_____

_____

_____

_____

_____

_____

The Pitfalls of Pain Management

Traditional pain management uses a multitude of interventions, including medications. Opioid medications are the primary drugs used to treat chronic pain and are often the cornerstone of pain management. Unfortunately, they carry with them a potential for side effects, decrease in function, and the development of dependence and addiction. The side effects of opioids may include cloudy thinking, drowsiness, depression, and sleep disturbance. In women, opioids and chronic pain can lower estrogen levels, even leading to early menopause and osteoporosis.

In some cases, increasing the dose of opioids can actually cause more pain, a phenomenon known as opioid-induced hyperalgesia (OIH) that occurs in some people who are on long-term opioids. The proper treatment of OIH is to discontinue opioid medications under medical supervision so the brain can "reset" and eliminate the hyperalgesic effect of the drugs.

It may amaze you to know that there are no scientifically reliable studies that justify the use of opioids for longer than three months, even though use of that length is standard operating procedure for treatment of chronic pain. There are a number of reasons for this disparity, but probably the best explanation is that opioids offer temporary relief to a permanent problem that is complex and difficult to treat. Doctors and drug companies have created an industry that promotes these powerful drugs for chronic pain, even though for many that is not the best course. Many people say they would never have started taking prescribed pain medication if they had known how much havoc it could wreak in their lives.

Additionally, as in Amy's case, painkillers are frequently prescribed in conjunction with other habit-forming medications, such as muscle relaxants (specifically Soma), stimulants used for sleepiness caused by the opioids, antianxiety drugs, and sleeping pills. The use of medications to treat the effects of other medications can be extremely frustrating for people with chronic pain and their families. Amy ended up on so many medications that her quality of life was severely compromised, and she still had significant pain. As a nurse, Mary certainly knew that Jim was no longer benefiting from his medications, but felt helpless to change anything. After all, "he's in pain and can't stop them," or so Jim told her whenever she brought it up.

Many medications are not habit-forming and may be prescribed as part of a pain management plan; these include muscle relaxants, antiseizure medicines, and antidepressants. Pain management also often includes invasive procedures such as injections (epidurals, facet blocks, and others) and surgeries, as well as nonmedication and nonsurgical techniques such as acupuncture, chiropractic, physical therapy, massage, and hydrotherapy.

Prescription Pain Medications

We've described potential problems with taking opioids for chronic pain. Here are the names of medications in this class and other classes of drugs with habit-forming potential:

Table 1.1a

Mood-altering & Potentially Addictive Drugs (This list is not all-inclusive.)			
Schedule	Type	Brand Name	Generic Name/Ingredients
II	Opioids	Actiq	Oral Transmucosal Fentanyl Citrate
II	Amphetamines	Adderal	Amphetamine Aspartate/Sulfate
IV	Diet	Adipex-P	Phentermine Tartrate
IV	Hypnotics (for sleep)	Ambien	Zolpidem Titrate
IV	Benzodiazepines	Ativan	Lorazepam
II	Opioids	Avinza	Morphine Sulfate
III	Diet	Bontril	Phentermine Tartrate
III	Antitussives and/or Expectorants	Brontex	Codeine Phosphate and Guiafenesin
II	Stimulants	Concerta	Methylphenidate
IV	Stimulants	Cylert	Pemoline
IV	Benzodiazepines	Dalmane	Flurazepam
IV	Opioids	Darvocet-N	Propoxyphene/Acetaminophen
IV	Opioids	Darvon	Propoxyphene
IV	Opioids	Darvon Compound	Propoxyphene/Aspirin/Caffeine
II	Opioids	Demerol	Meperidine
II	Amphetamines	Dexedrine	Dextroamphetamine
III	Diet	Didrex	Benzphetamine
II	Opioids	Dilaudid	Hydromorphone
IV	Benzodiazepines	Doral	Quazepam
II	Opioids	Duragesic	Fentanyl
IV	Muscle Relaxants	Equagesic	Meprobamate/Aspirin
III	Barbiturates	Fioricet/Codeine	Butalbital/Codeine/Acet/Caffeine
III	Barbiturates	Fiorinal	Butalbital/Aspirin/Caffeine
III	Barbiturates	Fiorinal/Codeine	Butalbital/Codeine/ASA/Caffeine
II	Stimulants	Focalin	Dexmethylphenidate
IV	Benzodiazepines	Halcion	Triazolam
III	Antitussives and/or Expectorants	Hycodan	Hydrocodone/Methylbromide
III	Antitussives and/or Expectorants	Hycotuss	Hydrocodone/Guiafenesin
IV	Diet	Ionamin	Phentermine Tartrate
II	Opioids	Kadian	Morphine Sulfate
IV	Benzodiazepines	Klonopin	Clonazepam
IV	Benzodiazepines	Librium	Chlordiazepoxide
III	Opioids	Lorcet	Hydrocodone/Acetaminophen

continued on page 13

Schedule	Type	Brand Name	Generic Name/Ingredients
		Mood-altering & Potentially Addictive Drugs (*continued*)	
III	Opioids	Lortab	Hydrocodone/Acetaminophen
IV	Hypnotics (for sleep)	Lunesta	Eszopiclone
III	Opioids	Maxidone	Hydrocodone/Acetaminophen
IV	Diet	Meridia	Sibutramine Monohydrate
II	Stimulants	Metadate	Methylphenidate
II	Opioids	Methadone	Methadone
II	Opioids	MS Contin	Morphine Sulfate
II	Opioids	MSIR	Morphine Sulfate
III	Opioids	Nucynta	Tapentadol
III	Opioids	Norco	Hydrocodone/Acetaminophen
II	Opioids	Oxycontin	Oxycodone
II	Opioids	Oxyfast	Oxycodone
II	Opioids	OxyIR	Oxycodone
III	Opioids	Panlor DC	Dihydrocodeine/Acet/Caffeine
II	Opioids	Percocet	Oxycodone/Acetaminophen
II	Opioids	Percodan	Oxycodone/Aspirin
IV	Barbiturates	Phenobarbital	Phenobarbital
III	Antitussives and/or Expectorants	Prolex DH	Hydrocodone Bitartrate Potassium
IV	Benzodiazepines	Prosom	Estazolam
IV	Antinarcoleptics	Provigil	Modafinil
IV	Benzodiazepines	Restoril	Temazepam
II	Stimulants	Ritalin	Methylphenidate
IV	Benzodiazepines	Serax	Oxazepam
III	Muscle Relaxants	Soma	Carisoprodol
III	Muscle Relaxants	Soma Compound	Carisoprodol/Aspirin/Codeine
IV	Hypnotics (for sleep)	Sonata	Zaleplon
IV	Opioids	Stadol NS	Butorphanol Tartrate
III	Opioids	Subutex/Suboxone	Buprenorphine Hydrochloride
III	Opioids	Synalgos DC	Dihydrocodeine Bitartrate/Caffeine
IV	Opioids	Talacen	Pentazocine/Acetaminophen
IV	Opioids	Talwin NX	Pentazocine Naloxone
IV	Diet	Tenuate	Diethylpropion
IV	Benzodiazepines	Tranxene	Clorazepate Dipotassium
III	Antitussive and/or Expectorants	Tussionex	Hydrocodone Bit/Chlorpheniramine
III	Opioids	Tylenol/Codeine	Acetaminophen/Codeine
IV	Nonopioid Painkiller	Ultram, Ultracet	Tramadol
II	Opioids	Tylox	Oxycodone/Acetaminophen
IV	Nonopioid Painkiller	Ultram, Ultracet	Tramadol
IV	Benzodiazepines	Valium	Diazepam
III	Opioids	Vicodin	Hydrocodone/Acetaminophen
III	Opioids	Vicoprofen	Hydrocodone/Ibuprofen
IV	Benzodiazepines	Xanax	Alprazolam
III	Opioids	Zydone	Hydrocodone/Acetaminophen

There are a number of nonopioid medications that are used to decrease pain. Here's a partial list:

Table 1.1b

Nonopioid Medications		
Drug Class		**Generic**	**Brand Name(s)**
Anticonvulsants		Gabapentin	Neurontin
		Topiramate	Topamax
		Carbemazepine	Tegretol
		Valproic Acid	Depakote
		Pregablin	Lyrica
Anti-depressants	**Tricyclics**	Amitryptilline	Elavil
		Desipramine	Norpramin
		Norpramine	Pamelor
	SSRI–SNRI	Venflaxine	Effexor
		Duloxetine	Cymbalta
NSAIDs	**COX 2s Traditional NSAIDs**	Celecoxib	Celebrex
		Ibuprofen	Advil, Motrin
		Naproxen	Naprosyn, Aleve
		Indomethacin	Indocin
		Nabunetone	Relafen
Muscle Relaxants		Methocarbamol	Robaxin
		Liorisal	Baclofen
		Metaxalone	Skelaxin
		Cyclobenzaprine	Flexeril
		Tizanadine	Xanaflex
Topicals		Capascins	Zostrix
		Lidocaine	Lidoderm patches Flector patches

{ *exercise* 1.5 }

_____'s *Pain Management Experience* _____

List the medications that have been prescribed for _____, as well as those he or she is using that are not prescribed (put a P next to those prescribed and an N next to those not prescribed). You can refer to the list in Tables 1.1(a) and 1.1(b).

_____

_____

_____

_____

_____

_____

_____

Now list any substances _____ has used in addition to medications.
Include alcohol, over-the-counter products, cigarettes, caffeine, and illegal drugs.

_____

_____

_____

_____

_____

_____

Finally, list any treatment modalities or procedures _____ has used or
undergone for pain management. Indicate "+" or "−" as to whether they were helpful
or not.

_____

_____

_____

_____

_____

_____

_____

*As you read this chapter, your mind may be churning with frustration, fear, anger, and
confusion. How did you get here, and what do you do now? Is there a way out? Indeed
there is, so read on and get ready to work. In the next chapter, you will see more clearly
how your life has become based on the well-being of your person with pain. And you
will begin to see how you can move toward balancing your own life, regardless of how
_____ is doing.*

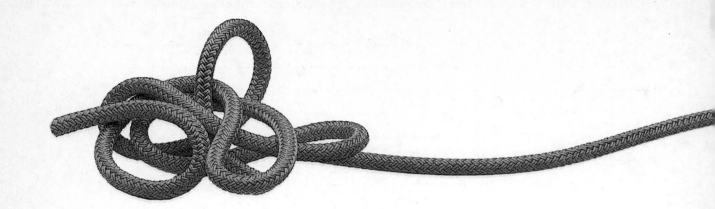

2

How Families React to Chronic Pain

After Jim's injury, he was laid up in the hospital for a while, then came home and hadn't worked since — over four years ago. He couldn't sit up or concentrate long enough even to do therapy. He was severely depressed and in pain twenty-four/seven. Two surgeries and countless epidural injections had left him no better, and, in fact, worse after the last surgery; now he had burning and tingling down his right leg that kept him from resting, so he was up and down all night. Mary nursed Jim in the hospital and at home for as long as she could, but finally money was running out and she was compelled to return to work. At the time, she still had one of her kids at home, whom she felt she was abandoning because she had to leave to work nights as a nurse at a local hospital. It was actually a relief to be out of the house (though she hated herself for feeling it). At least she could care for people who got better. And she didn't have to live with them — with their pain, their complaining, their depression, and their anger. At home, that's mostly what dominated her life and the life of her family. Jim tried his best, but it seemed like his best wasn't nearly enough. The pain was getting the best of him, and driving them both, not to mention the kids, crazy!

Thankfully, Mandi was out of the house, recently graduating from college and going on to graduate school. She wanted to help, even offering to quit school and return home, but Mary categorically refused. The last thing she wanted was for her successful daughter to get sucked into the downward spiral that had become their life. Ross had become more sullen and withdrawn lately. Mary was sure he was missing his dad. They were both subject to Jim's moodiness — one minute shouting, the next crying. Mary knew it was taking its toll on her teenaged son and didn't know where to turn.

When chronic pain is introduced into the family, everything changes. Along with these changes, a variety of confusing and negative emotions often develop as the whole family is thrown off balance by role reversals, medical concerns, financial and legal worries, and other lifestyle shifts. It can be difficult for even a well-functioning family to adapt in a positive way; in fact, it is uncommon to see a healthy adjustment to such a trauma.

While every family's experience is unique, there tends to be a pattern to how families respond to chronic pain, which may occur rapidly or over a long period of time. When a member of the family becomes disabled by chronic pain, the rest of the family steps up and takes on more responsibilities. These responsibilities can include earning money for the family, doing household chores, caring for children, and any other functions the person in pain fulfilled in the past but is now unable to fulfill. As family roles change, each person's sense of self has to readjust. Mary had stopped working as a nurse to become a full-time mom, and all of a sudden she had to figure out how to earn a living for the family when Jim could no longer work. Jim's pain changed his identity as the breadwinner, and also caused him to be absent from activities he enjoyed with the kids—soccer practice, helping them study, etc.

With the role shifts, everybody suffers an incremental loss as a little bit is chipped away from their sense of self and the part of them that was defined by their relationship with the person in pain.

A shift you may have experienced is that suddenly _____ has become the central figure in your life, with everyone else revolving around him or her: running, getting, doing, trying to make things better, compensating for, and trying to fill the vacancies. This can leave you with little time to take care of or enjoy yourself. You may be feeling resentful or depressed, but you may believe that these feelings are inappropriate because you are not the one in pain. You have become less interested in your own needs, because _____ is the one who needs attention.

Mary's role as Jim's caretaker eventually became her primary identity. This continuous sacrificing of her own needs to the needs of another led to her feeling overwhelmed by feelings of anger, sadness, and guilt, which began negatively affecting her own health.

Often with chronic pain, everyone in the family system feels like they're carrying a burden. Everyone feels victimized by the pain, but may not be communicating their feelings to each other or seeking support to help them cope, at a time when they need support the most.

Am I Out of Balance? _____

Please answer "Yes" or "No" to the following questions. Fill in the blanks with the name of your family member who has chronic pain.

Yes	No	Does your life revolve around _____?
Yes	No	Is your well-being dependent on _____'s well-being?
Yes	No	If _____ hurts, do you hurt, or are you unable to have fun, concentrate on your work, or take proper care of yourself or others in your life?
Yes	No	Do you feel guilty when you are impatient, annoyed, or simply not there?
Yes	No	Is your life spinning out of control in your attempts to help?
Yes	No	Are you depressed, angry, fearful, anxious, irritable?
Yes	No	Are you unable to see any way out of these emotions?

If the answer to any of these questions is "Yes," then this chapter will help frame the problem and suggest the beginnings of some solutions for you and ultimately the people who are important to you, including _____.

Taking a Family Systems Approach

Describing the family as a *system* helps us to better understand the effects of chronic pain on the family as a whole, rather than on each member individually. In a family systems approach, what is important is looking at the family as a functioning unit, in terms of how the actions of each family member affects the rest of the family, both individually and as a whole. Thus, when _____ developed chronic pain, that change in him or her naturally had effects on every member of the family and on the way the family operates (e.g., interacts or communicates). However, in a family systems approach, your actions and reactions will also affect the family, including _____.

FAMILY SYSTEMS: A BRIEF INTRODUCTION

While a complete discussion of the many different family systems theories is beyond the scope of this book, a brief discussion of the central ideas common to all of them will be presented here. Reviewing this brief discussion will help you to understand what is going on in your family and how it could be changed.

From a systems perspective, a family is considered to be a system whose members are interdependent. This means that each member of the family can function independently, but they also turn to one another for support and can have effects on one another. Each family can also have several subsystems that have generational links and boundaries, communication networks, coalitions and alliances, rules, secrets, myths, and rituals.

The important or key dimensions and terms include:

1. **Adaptability:** whether the family is flexible, as opposed to chaotic or rigid, in its functioning and its ability to adapt in order to effectively handle problems as they arise.

2. **Cohesion:** to what degree the family sticks together and is interdependent, as opposed to being disengaged (i.e., too cut off) from each other or enmeshed (i.e., in each other's business, codependent, or enabling).

3. **Family Communication:** how well the family communicates with each other, which can facilitate their adaptability and cohesiveness.

4. **Dynamics:** how the system interacts, including patterns and the effects of one's actions on the rest of the system and individual members.

5. **Interaction Patterns:** related to dynamics. This is how the family members interact with each other. Boundaries, family rules and roles, and nonverbal behavior (e.g., whether closed doors are respected) are important here.

   Interaction patterns can involve triangles (a third person intervening to referee a conflict), stable coalitions (two members repeatedly aligned against a third), detouring coalitions (two agree on identifying a third as the source of the problem, which can give others an impression of harmony), triangulation (two members both insist that a third member side with him or her), and splitting (playing two people against each other). In the triangulation scenario, the third member asked to be aligned with two others may develop symptomatic behavior as a result of the conflict of being pulled in two different directions. Boundaries are important here as well (as they are in cohesiveness), and can be either too rigid (blocks interaction between members) or enmeshed (overly open, in each other's business, codependent, or enabling).

6. **Homeostasis:** what a family system does to keep functioning "normally"—in the same way it has always functioned, for better or worse (i.e., functional or dysfunctional). For example, dysfunctional families often work hard to keep family secrets from being revealed by creating unspoken rules such as "Don't ask; don't tell."

Thus, a healthy family system is one that is flexible or adaptable, has a well-defined structure, and is cohesive. Healthy families can therefore accommodate changes in the roles and functions of individual members, family subsystems, and the entire family unit. Also, healthy families can accommodate changes within the sociocultural context. By contrast, dysfunctional families have a limited capacity to cope effectively because of rigidity or chaos in their functioning and structure, unhealthy alliances and power balances within the system, and persistent boundary problems.

Before Jim's injury, he was the breadwinner, Mary was the mom and homemaker, and the kids were unruly teenagers. Their level of adaptability was limited, and much chaos ensued in the family system after Jim was hurt. Their communication skills were limited, so they couldn't make sense of the enormous changes. Most of the family rules in that household were unspoken, and after a while no one talked with anyone about what was occurring. Mandi escaped from the environment with relief when she went off to college. Ross started using pot, and his grades dropped. Mary could barely keep her head above water, and just let it happen; she felt she had no choice.

As Amy became less functional, Chris became more and more isolated—from her and from others. He was terribly embarrassed by Amy's limitations and behaviors, so he stopped calling and interacting with friends. Whereas previously they were a balanced, self-assured couple, the two of them became more enmeshed, and because of her progressive drug dependence, she became totally dependent on him for any support.

Identifying Effects of Chronic Pain on Your Family System _____ { *exercise* 2.2 }

1. Describe your family's functioning in terms of the following (refer to the definitions provided in the previous section):

ADAPTABILITY
(Circle the word that best describes how adaptable your family is.)

Rigid   Flexible   Chaotic

COHESIVENESS
(Circle the word that best describes how well you stick together.)

Disconnected   Interdependent   Enmeshed/Codependent

INTERACTION PATTERNS
(Are there any of the following?)

Triangles   Coalitions   Triangulation   Splitting

BOUNDARIES

(Circle the word that best describes how boundaries are within your family.)

Rigid   Flexible   Chaotic   Nonexistent

FAMILY ROLES

(Describe the roles that each of your family members plays.)

_____

_____

_____

_____

_____

_____

FAMILY RULES

(Describe any rules that control the actions of family members. How have the rules changed?)

_____

_____

_____

_____

_____

_____

2. Describe how the family responded when _____ was first injured or developed pain problems.

_____

_____

_____

_____

_____

_____

3. As _____'s pain became chronic or unchanging, how did the family seem to respond?

_____

_____

_____

_____

_____

_____

4. Comparing how things are now (refer to your answers to the first question in this exercise) to how your family functioned before the onset of _____'s chronic pain problems, describe the most noticeable differences.

_____

_____

_____

_____

_____

_____

Codependent and Enabling Behaviors

Most people have heard the term "codependence." Codependence originally referred to an addict being dependent on drugs, and the partner in the relationship being dependent on the addict, and thus codependent. However, codependency is not just a characteristic of addiction. Codependence is a cluster of behaviors that often occurs in people affected by an addicted person's behavior. Thus, codependence occurs in relationships and can be defined as one person's tendency to be overly focused or centered on another rather than on him- or herself. Typically, the codependent person feels compelled to meet the needs of other people, to fix or control others (e.g., the addict). Because of this unhealthy desire to meet the needs of the other person in the relationship, the codependent person can become the *enabler* of the other person's addictive behavior. Additionally, the codependent person protects the other person from the natural consequences of the addictive behavior. For example, a codependent person may not mention, pretend not to notice, or make excuses (e.g., "He's just tired.") for obvious signs of intoxication in his or her partner, despite how angry he or she feels. This denial enables the addictive behavior, making it seem acceptable via the silence, and also protects the addict from being confronted about the behavior.

Codependence can affect any relationship, not just those involving a drug-dependent person. For people with codependent tendencies, being in a relationship that requires taking care of someone (e.g., a person with chronic pain) is a perfect scenario for codependency to flourish. For example, in relationships involving a person with chronic pain, a spouse may enable his or her spouse's isolation and withdrawal from the family by not confronting him or her about it. As a codependent person, you may unknowingly enable and contribute to your partner's continued imbalance (addiction, chronic pain, etc.). Enabling allows this pattern to continue in an unhealthy fashion.

It should be noted that this discussion of codependence barely scratches the surface of a very important and complicated topic. There are many good information sources available for further reading on codependence, including *Choicemaking: For Spirituality Seekers, Codependents and Adult Children* by Sharon Wegscheider-Cruse (HCI); *Adult Children: The Secrets of Dysfunctional Families* by John and Linda Friel (HCI); and *Codependent No More: How to Stop Controlling Others and Start Caring for Yourself* by Melody Beattie (Hazelden).

Mary enabled Jim's isolation and withdrawal from the family by not confronting him and not communicating how upsetting his behavior was. When Amy didn't get out of bed for a week, Chris began feeding her in bed. His intention was to take care of her and to prevent her from starving; but when he feeds her in bed, she doesn't have to get out of bed. He is reinforcing her pain, and she has become more and more dependent on him. This contributes to his sense of powerlessness and unmanageability.

Enabling involves not being able to set appropriate boundaries. Boundaries become distorted when family members begin to take over responsibilities that the person in pain is capable of handling for him- or herself. This is usually driven by guilt and a desire to make up for the situation the person in pain is in. The enabling behavior is the natural response of the caretaker to the afflicted loved one, but instead of helping, it creates an unhealthy dependency and prevents the person in pain from maintaining self-sufficiency, which reinforces pain and helplessness. Family members often enable the person in pain to engage in victim thinking and behavior.

Identifying Codependency in You and _____ _____

This exercise will help you to identify codependent traits in yourself and in _____. Read the following list of characteristics and indicate which apply to you, to _____, or to both of you (check both boxes).

Self	Other Person	Characteristic
		Problems trusting others (anticipating betrayal), making true intimacy very difficult.
		"People-pleasing," an excessive need or desire to do what other people want, often at the expense of one's own needs.
		Covering or making excuses for behavior so as to avoid having to deal with the consequences, e.g., telling family that someone is "sick" or "tired" when he or she has taken too much pain medication or is drunk.
		A need to be in control of self.
		A need to be in control of others.
		Always depending on another for guidance.
		Discounting or doubting one's own judgment.
		Always being worried about making the wrong decision.
		Ending up in relationships with people who need to be taken care of.
		Ending up in relationships with people who initially need help, but later take advantage or become abusive in some way.
		Fear of feeling angry (i.e., losing control), to the point of avoiding confrontation or conflict and/or denying that you are angry.
		Lying, omitting information, or exaggerating, even when it would be easier to tell the truth.
		Fearing abandonment.
		Fear of being alone.
		Tolerating hurtful behaviors.
		Guilt about not being able to take away the pain.
		Guilt for being angry.

THE SOLICITOUS SPOUSE

Research has shown that in the presence of a "solicitous spouse" (one who genuinely cares and expresses concern), pain and disability increase. Studies on chronic pain sufferers found that when their spouses focused more attention on the pain problem and engaged in overlyprotective, solicitous behaviors, their reported pain and degree of disability increased. Solicitous behaviors can include asking repeatedly if the person is in pain, suggesting that he or she lie down, or asking if the person has taken his or her pain medication. When the spouse paid less attention to the pain problem or actively tried to get the chronic pain sufferer to focus on other things, his or her reported pain and degree of disability decreased. Though this research focused on the spouse, what it illustrates is that if you reinforce pain (through codependent and enabling behaviors), the pain is maintained.

Mary's tendency was to stroke Jim's brow when he complained of pain. She'd coddle him and even use baby talk at times in an attempt to soothe his discomfort. This reinforcing behavior actually caused him to report and to feel more pain than when Mary was at work and he had to do for himself. He developed a lack of the ability to self-soothe. Sometimes, without realizing it, he groaned and complained to evoke a response from her. Imagine what would happen when she failed to respond the first time, being distracted, exhausted, or just annoyed. This became a source of great friction for them.

THE COMPASSIONATE BRAIN

We also know that our brains are wired to react empathetically when someone else is in pain. A study was conducted where people were shown videos of a person experiencing pain. Brain scans revealed that the same areas of the brain "light up" in the person who is watching someone in pain as in the person who is experiencing the pain. Literally, we feel another's pain. And this empathetic reaction is much stronger when the person in pain is a family member. So it is only natural to develop enabling behaviors when a loved one is in pain. It is our innate response to feel another's pain and to want to do something to help, but it is just those solicitous or enabling behaviors that make the pain worse.

Reinforcing pain causes more pain; reinforcing function enhances function.

When Amy cried with her pain, it would break Chris's heart. He didn't think he could stand it. He often gave her medication before it was due (he had confiscated her medications in an attempt to control her drug use), even though she appeared to be "loaded." He simply couldn't tolerate the feelings that came up when he witnessed her suffering. What would happen if he didn't give her the meds? He didn't want to find out.

Enabling Responses _____

You may be unknowingly responding to _____'s pain in ways that make the pain worse. This exercise will help you identify ways in which this may be occurring.

Please complete the following sentences with the *first response* that comes to mind.

1. I can tell when _____ is in more pain because

_____

_____.

2. When I know his or her pain is getting worse, I usually

_____

_____.

3. When it's time for _____ to take more pain medication, I usually

_____

_____.

4. If _____ tells me he or she is hurting more, I tell him or her

_____

_____.

5. If I want to go out to dinner or some other activity and _____ says he or she is in too much pain to go, I usually

_____

_____.

Secondary Gain: A Hidden Obstacle to Recovery

Secondary gain is a psychiatric term that means any hidden reason that is motivating a person to hold onto an undesirable condition or problematic behavior. Here it can refer to any perceived benefit _____ receives from having pain, or it can refer to any perceived benefit you receive from _____'s pain. If not identified, secondary gain can cause you to unconsciously hold onto unhealthy behaviors. This does not mean _____ is pretending to hurt for these benefits, or that you want him or her to remain in pain, just that the benefits are making the pain rewarding in some ways and thus more complicated to treat.

Some examples of secondary gain that might result from having chronic pain are listed below. Check those that apply to _____.

_____ Receiving more attention.

_____ Not having to work.

_____ Being excused from responsibilities.

_____ Being on disability—essentially, being paid to be in pain.

_____ Getting out of activities.

_____ Having an excuse to take pills.

Some examples of secondary gain that might result from caring for someone with chronic pain are listed below. Check those that apply to you.

_____ Giving you a sense of purpose and meaning in life.

_____ Being the hero/caregiver/helper/rescuer (having someone who rewards your need to be needed).

_____ Being able to "people please."

_____ Being in more control or having more power in the household.

_____ Getting you out of the house, since you have to work to support family.

_____ Being the major breadwinner.

_____ Receiving disability benefits that help support the family.

_____ Expecting a large financial windfall from a lawsuit due to injuries.

_____ Reinforcing your sense of being a martyr/victim, fulfilling a need from early childhood.

When you become aware of them, you may view secondary gain as deserved compensation for the challenges you are experiencing. These thought processes may be conscious but are usually totally unconscious. Either way, if these beliefs remain unexamined, they will interfere with your ability to improve your situation. Taking inventory of secondary gain you and _____ may be experiencing, and examining your attitudes about this, is an important step in moving toward balance.

Identifying Secondary Gain _____

{ *exercise* }
2.5

List all the real and perceived benefits you have ever received from _____ having chronic pain. Be sure to include the things you get, as well as things you were or are able to avoid. One example of each is provided for thought.

PHYSICAL ___

{example: I do not have to be involved in activities I never really liked because _____ can't do them now.}

MENTAL ___

{example: Since _____ is out of it most of the time, I can speak my mind more freely.}

EMOTIONAL ___

{example: I can avoid emotional intimacy.}

FAMILIAL ___

(Include emotional as well as specific household or practical responsibilities.)
{example: I am in charge of what happens around here.}

SOCIAL/WORK LIFE

{example: Just like I always wanted, I have to go to work. What a relief!}

SEXUAL

{example: He's in too much pain for physical intimacy, so I don't have to do that anymore.}

It's important to look closely at secondary gain, as the perceived benefits might not be as attractive as you believe. Most of the time secondary gain is not gain at all, but loss. Chronic pain sufferers and their families often inadvertently buy into the concept of secondary gain without looking at primary loss.

{ *exercise* 2.6 }

Examining Secondary Gain _____

Go over the list of examples of secondary gain you identified and take a minute to look at what is actually going on. Write about your observations.

_____
_____
_____
_____
_____
_____

Most people find they are just stuck and afraid to move forward. Once you walk through this fear, you will find you gain much more by a return to normalcy in your life.

Looking back, Chris couldn't say exactly when things had changed for Amy and him, but it was probably soon after she started on Lortab and Soma for the diffuse pain all over her body that left her anxious and depressed. When she started taking the pills, everything got better for both of them for a while because Amy's pain was reduced, but eventually the doses and strength of the pills increased. The pain doctor she found had rapidly advanced her medication intake. She became emotionally distant; she seemed to disappear into a drug haze, but when unmedicated, she was miserable with the pain. Chris called her doctor to discuss his concerns but was unable to speak with anyone because of HIPAA* restrictions. Amy was clearly addicted to her medications, which became a complicating factor in her relationship with Chris. Chris now had to deal with his responses to chronic pain as well as her addiction.

In this chapter, we've discussed the many ways in which families react to the entry of chronic pain into the system and how it can upset the balance of the family system. Important in this discussion are the issues of what defines a family system and the effects that chronic pain has had on your family, as well as codependence, enabling, and secondary gain. We hope you have seen how these issues relate to you and your family. With this background, we turn now to a discussion of addiction and the effects of drugs on the family.

The **Health Insurance Portability and Accountability Act (HIPAA) provides federal protections for personal health information held by covered entities and gives patients an array of rights with respect to that information.*

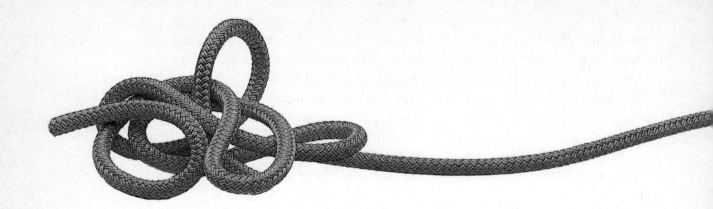

3

Chronic Pain and Addiction: Double Trouble

During a rare moment of clarity, Amy admitted to herself that her life was a mess. She had deteriorated over the last few years, experiencing increasing pain and a general feeling of being a loser—and the more drugs she took, the worse she got. On some level she knew her screwed-up life was caused by the drugs she was taking, though she'd deny that to Chris with a vengeance. That usually shut him up, but lately it was getting tougher, and he was more verbal, more critical, and more demanding.

Deep down Amy knew she was destined to become addicted. After all, both of her parents were; her dad died of a heroin overdose, and her mom was addicted to hydrocodone, OxyContin, morphine, and valium—the same meds she was taking. So it was inevitable from her first dose of codeine cough syrup she took as an adolescent. These drugs "worked" in her brain. They made her feel like she could cope better with the world and, lately, Chris. She reflected on the irony of her developing addiction, similar to her family's, although she had vowed, "It will never happen to me." It was as if the drugs carried her away, or took control, robbing her of her free will.

According to a 2006 study, 90 percent of all people in the United States receiving treatment for pain management receive prescriptions for opioid medication, like both Jim and Amy did. These medications carry with them a risk of dependency and addiction. For those with chronic pain who become addicted when they take opioids for pain relief, the two conditions exacerbate each other, making both worse than they would be alone. Many professionals believe the benefits of opioid treatment far outweigh the risk of developing addiction, but those who do become addicted find themselves in a conundrum: They need opioids to treat pain, but when they take them, they experience horrible consequences. This presents a huge dilemma for those of you in Mary's or Chris's position.

Addiction Explained

Addiction is a complex brain disease. The symptoms of addiction include physical, emotional, spiritual, and thought disturbances, with manifestations that affect behaviors and relationships. Use of drugs over time induces changes in the structure and function of the brain that can be long-lasting and produce a host of harmful effects. Studies have shown that in drug-addicted individuals, the areas of the brain that undergo physical changes are critical to judgment, decision making, emotion, memory, and behavior control. This may help explain the destructive behaviors of addiction. As the disease progresses, a person becomes increasingly unable to control his or her drug seeking and use even in the face of terrible consequences.

Amy had tried drugs early; she had smoked pot for the first time at age twelve. That and the fact that both of her parents had addiction increased her chances of developing it. People who have a family history of addiction or a history of addiction themselves are at much higher risk for developing problems with painkillers. The best solution would be for those people to never start those medications; however, some people will choose to take painkillers, find a doctor who insists on them, or inadvertently end up taking them. Although there is no way to predict with certainty whether a person will become addicted to drugs, there are several known risk factors. These include:

Genes: It is estimated that genetics accounts for at least 40 to 60 percent of a person's vulnerability to addiction.

Environment: Frequent exposure to drug use in home, work, school, or social life can influence a person's use of drugs, which may become problematic.

Early use of drugs: The earlier a person starts using drugs, the more likely he or she is to develop problems with abuse and addiction.

Mental illness: Anxiety, depression, and other mood disorders are commonly associated with addiction.

Traumatic childhood experiences: Abuse, neglect, dysfunction in the family, or other trauma can leave a child more susceptible to addiction later in life.

When Amy entered therapy a few years later, she realized she had been suppressing memories of sexual fondling by her babysitter when she was a little girl.

Addiction is a chronic, relapsing brain disease characterized by compulsive drug seeking and use, despite harmful consequences. At one time, addiction was a pharmacologic term that referred to a person's using enough drugs to cause tolerance and physical dependence. In fact, we now know a person can have addiction without developing tolerance or physical dependence.

Tolerance means that more of the drug is needed over time to experience the same effect, and it commonly occurs with long-term use of opioids.

Physical dependence is characterized by being unable to stop using the drug without feeling terrible and developing a syndrome known as withdrawal.

Drug dependence is a synonym for addiction and is a set of behaviors involving problematic use of mood-altering substances over a continuous period of time.

Amy had the following symptoms of drug (opioid) dependence:

- She had problems with *controlling* use, and thus had an unpredictable outcome once she began using a substance. She was overusing her prescription medications, needing to supplement her medication supply from "friends."

- Because of pressure from Chris she tried to *cut down*, and once even quit for a few days, but she was unable to "stay stopped."

- She was *preoccupied* with the drug, focusing on the clock, waiting for her next dose.

- She *continued to use* the drugs even though her use was ruining her relationship with Chris and causing her work to suffer miserably.

- She *stopped doing the things she used to do*, like bowling and needlepoint.

- She spent *more and more time "chasing the high"* — spending time and energy going to multiple doctors to get the drugs. When she had an ample supply, she would overuse and then lose days at a time, being high and in bed.

With addiction, the problem exists not so much with the drug itself as with the way that drug works in Amy's brain and nervous system. Amy was destined to develop addiction because of how "well" drugs worked in her brain — both physically and emotionally. She was probably wired differently from birth, inheriting addiction from both of her parents. With continued exposure to the drug, particularly the opioids (whether she started taking them for pain or not), she eventually became addicted.

Jim and Amy both developed tolerance and physical dependence. These phenomena occur with continued exposure to certain substances over time. With increased use of certain drugs (e.g., an opioid), the body reacts by decreasing the effect of the drug, in this case pain relief. This is tolerance. Consequently, in order to achieve pain relief, Jim and Amy increased the dose of the drugs they were taking. This adjustment worked temporarily, but eventually the need for still-increased doses occurred. Eventually, the drug seemed not to work any longer, which resulted in using stronger, more potent drugs in an escalating upward spiral.

As Jim and Amy became tolerant to their medications, their bodies were "normalized" in the presence of the drugs. In fact, they became so used to the drug that they *needed* the drug to feel normal. Without it, they felt terrible. This is physical dependence. When the drugs are discontinued abruptly, they feel withdrawal—in effect, the opposite feelings that the drug caused. So if opioids cause decreased pain and some amount of calmness and well-being, then withdrawal consists of increased pain and anxiety, body aches, stomach and muscle cramps, diarrhea, nausea, vomiting, insomnia, and agitation. This outcome is one of the main reasons people will feel the need to continue the opioid, since, when they try to stop or even reduce the dose, they feel terrible.

What is the solution to this awful problem? Jim and Amy felt that they had to take drugs to feel any level of pain relief, even though the drugs were barely working. In fact, they actually may have been making the pain worse due to opioid-induced hyperalgesia. Jim considered cutting down the dose of the opioid; however, that presented the immediate problem of withdrawal. In the short run, cutting down or stopping made him feel much worse. This is because the withdrawal of the opioid from his system inevitably caused a temporary increase in symptoms, including pain. This effect made the process of coming off opioids challenging, but not impossible for Jim. He and his doctor decided to substitute one opioid for another, which temporarily put off the process, but proved not to solve anything.

Addiction is a chronic disease similar to other chronic diseases such as type II diabetes, cancer, and cardiovascular disease.
–National Institute on Drug Abuse

We have treated hundreds of people like Jim and Amy, who are tolerant to and dependent on opioids. The withdrawal from these drugs is best done under medical supervision, and temporarily, patients typically feel worse. But on the other side, when the opioids have left their systems for a week or two, their pain diminishes and they start to feel better. The discomfort of withdrawal may continue for a while, even for several months in some, but eventually their nervous systems readjust to the absence of opioids and they return to a state of well-being that has escaped many of them for years. Meanwhile, as _____'s system heals, it will be helpful for you as a family member to begin the healing process as well.

Four Stages of Addiction

As with many illnesses, to understand the progressive nature of the disease of addiction, we have broken it down into stages. People who have addiction started in stage I and will inevitably end up in stage IV if not treated. The progression from stage I to IV may occur rapidly or may take years or decades. Stopping drug use might halt the disease process, but the disease is still present. Further, if use is restarted, the disease process will pick up where it left off. Like a train traveling from New York to California, if a user gets off in Chicago (stage II), the user will "reboard" in Chicago and continue west, heading inevitably toward stage IV, disability, and eventually death. Here are the stages in further detail:

Stages of Addiction

PROGRESSION OF DISEASE

STAGE 1	STAGE 2	STAGE 3	STAGE 4
First ingestion of substance	Deterioration of function; negative consequences	Intense desire for mood-changing effects	Late-stage: effects on all areas of life
SIGNS INCLUDE	SIGNS INCLUDE	SIGNS INCLUDE	SIGNS INCLUDE
Pain goes away	Problems in one of four areas:	Daily drug use, increasing doses	Multiple areas of problems
Craving	Home life/Family	Depression, maybe suicidal	Family/ Relationships gone
Counting pills	Job/School	Family problems/Divorce	Out of work/ School failure
Worrying if supply is low	Social function	Legal problems/ Arrested	Thinking impaired by drugs
Focusing on next dose	Legal/ Health status	Financial problems/Job loss	Needing more drugs to feel normal
Developing tolerance		Physical changes	Health consequences: brain dysfunction/ liver failure/ heart problems
Using for other purposes		Drug dependence, physical	
Adding other substances		Withdrawal symptoms	Overdoses common
Using stimulants for fatigue		Long-term chronic pain	

STAGE I

Stage I addiction begins with the first ingestion of a mood-altering drug. The feelings that occur are related to mood change. For Amy, it started with the first time she smoked marijuana as a teenager and it offered her a sense of "normalizing" the world, euphoria, and an energized sense of well-being. This sensation is especially true of the first use of opioid painkillers. The pain goes away—both the physical and the emotional pain. Although there may be no outward behavioral changes yet, such drug use cannot be considered "safe" because in people with the neurobiological risk for developing addiction, subsequent use may result in substance abuse and life changes beyond the person's control.

When they first started dating, Amy was in stage I. Chris had a greater awareness of the problematic use of substances than Amy. She had a nagging, uneasy sense that there was something wrong, but denied it to herself and to Chris. Amy tried to cut down and even quit using marijuana and cocaine for periods of time, but without recovery or treatment, typically she eventually resumed use and the problems recurred and escalated. When she was diagnosed with fibromyalgia and her pain started to escalate, things changed and she started abusing opioids.

Amy, who had both chronic pain and addiction, was defensive about her drug use and answered any criticism or questions about it by rationalizing, for example:

- Explaining why drug use is necessary: "I have to take these medicines for the pain so I can function," or "The doctor said I need to take this."

- Minimizing the consequences of drug use: "It's not that bad because I'm not taking that many," or "I only take what's prescribed and sometimes less" (hoarding extras "just in case"), or "I go to work every day, so I can't have a problem."

- Denying: "I don't have a problem with drugs."

Other characteristics of stage I may include:

- Wanting the drug (craving).

- Counting pills.

- Worrying when the supply of pills is low.

- Focusing on the time until the next dose (preoccupation).

- Increasing the dose without a doctor's order (tolerance).

- Taking a pill or two in the morning to "get going" (using for purposes other than those intended by the prescriber).

- Adding another substance to supplement the effects (commonly alcohol or other sedatives).

- Using stimulants because of fatigue caused by the opioids.

This stage usually occurs in individuals who haven't had chronic pain for long but are beginning to develop problems with opioids. For Amy, the pain worsened and so did her drug use. She progressed to stage II and then stage III rather quickly.

STAGE II

In stage II, Amy began to experience the negative consequences of drug use. This stage is characterized by problems in one of the following major functional areas: family or home life, job or school function, social function, legal status, or health. In stage II, people experience problems in one of these areas, although several areas may be affected as time goes on. Examples of stage II problems include:

- Fighting at home, neglecting familial responsibilities, or separation.

- Being disciplined at work or having decreased work performance.

- Calling in sick frequently or missing work without calling.

- Failing a major test at school or dropping classes.

- Using illegal methods to obtain drugs (consulting other doctors but not disclosing this to each doctor, acquiring pills from illegal sources, using multiple doctors or pharmacies, driving under the influence), but not yet having been caught or arrested.

- Experiencing a worsening of health problems, many of which are side effects of opioids, such as escalating pain, nausea, constipation, diarrhea, headaches, sleep disturbance, fatigue, or depression.

This stage usually occurs in individuals who have been dealing with chronic pain for some time, and though they may appear okay on the outside, they are beginning to experience deterioration of function.

For Amy, it was evidenced by frequent arguments and estrangement from Chris. Her work suffered and she started purchasing pills from "friends" at work, which of course was illegal.

STAGE III

In this stage, there is intense preoccupation with the desire to experience mood-changing effects of the drug(s). Daily drug use, depression, and thoughts of suicide are common. Family troubles increase. Legal problems may ensue. Stage III is characterized by any one of the following major consequences in any one major functional area. If family function is the problem area, these consequences include:

- Being asked to move out for good, leading to the end of the relationship.

- Getting a divorce.

- Becoming estranged from close family members.

If the problem areas are outside the home, they could include any of the following:

- Getting fired.

- Failing out of school.

- Going to jail.

Stage III physical changes include:

- Being hospitalized.

- Being physically dependent on drugs; suffering withdrawal when trying to cut down or stop.

To be considered stage III, the addict need have only one of these problems, not multiple problems in all areas of his or her life, even though that may be the case. This stage usually occurs in individuals who have been dealing with chronic pain for years, and the amount and variety of their medications have steadily increased, with progressive decrease in function, dependence on the drug(s), and general worsening of quality of life.

Amy entered stage III when she was fired from her job, and the next week she was arrested for buying drugs from an undercover narcotics officer.

STAGE IV

Stage IV is considered late-stage addiction, where the effects of the disease have spread to all areas of the person's life. Stage IV addiction, like stage IV cancer, is the period that precedes death from the disease. The length of time people can survive in this stage varies, but if the disease is treated, even at this point, the destructive process stops, life expectancy increases, and quality of life improves. Common causes of death from addiction include overdose, liver failure, accidents, suicide, and infections that would be preventable or treatable in nonaddicts. Those who have reached this stage need increasing quantities of drugs just to feel normal. Physical signs, such as damage to the heart, liver, and brain; malnutrition; lower resistance to pneumonia or tuberculosis; and overdoses are common.

Stage IV addiction is characterized by multiple problems in more than one major life area. Generally it means the person has no meaningful family life or relationships left, has no job or school life, is cognitively impaired by drug use, and has severe long-term, often permanent health consequences, including brain dysfunction. In stage IV, pain and addiction are deeply entrenched in a person's life and the person is alienated from loved ones and medical professionals alike. People with stage IV addiction fit the stereotype of those with addiction and are commonly homeless, in jail, or in an institution.

Individuals with chronic pain often have histories of overdosing on drugs, either accidentally or on purpose. The acetaminophen in their opioid medications has caused liver damage. Their lives consist of unending pain, periods of sleeping and sleeplessness, staying in bed most of the time, and trips to the emergency room, either to try to get drugs or for treatment of complications of the advanced disease.

*Considering Addiction*_____

{ *exercise* }
3.1

Do you think addiction is a disease? Why or why not?

_____
_____
_____
_____

Do you think _____ is an addict? Why or why not?

_____
_____
_____
_____

If yes, what stage is _____ in? Why do you think this? (List evidence.)

_____
_____
_____
_____

Neither Amy nor Jim had entered stage IV yet, but Amy wasn't too far from it. The high dose of acetaminophen in her painkillers was taking its toll. Chris's responses advanced in a similar fashion, going from concern to fear and annoyance, and finally to feeling fed up and ready to get out. Mary held fast as wife and chief enabler. Though her fuse was smoldering, it was still burning slowly and steadily. Unlike Chris, she couldn't conceive of getting out of the relationship, but she couldn't deny that the thoughts came up from time to time.

Regardless of which stage a person is in, the basic solution is the same, and treatment works. But the earlier, the better. As with any chronic disease, better treatment options exist before the disease has spread to all parts of the body. If the disease has progressed, which is often the case with chronic pain and addiction, more-involved and longer-term treatment may be necessary. It is best to consult with a professional who is familiar with co-occurring chronic pain and addiction.

Now that we have explained addiction, in the next chapter we would like to help you address your concerns about _____'s use of pain medications. We'll explore, in some depth, the reluctance, perhaps even overwhelming fear, that many people have about addiction and the term "addict." We will not tell you whether or not _____ is an addict, but we will provide you with facts so that you can make an accurate and informed assessment.

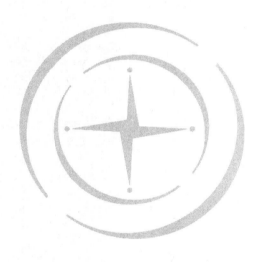

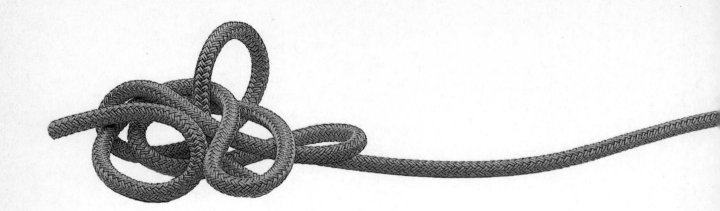

4

Is It Addiction?

Mary began to get concerned about Jim's use of medications, which included potent painkillers, muscle relaxers, and sleeping pills, with an occasional nerve pill thrown in. Thankfully, he wasn't drinking anymore, seeing the potential dangers of mixing alcohol with his medications. But the medications alone were making him loopy and dysfunctional. They frequently argued about Jim's use of drugs, especially since Mary had returned to nursing and was exposed to patients with drug overuse and abuse. He would always return to the fact that "I only take the drugs because I'm hurting. If I didn't have this damn pain, do you think I would continue to take them?" One day he shouted at her, "Are you calling me an addict?" when she pointed out that his dose had jumped in the last few months and didn't seem to be helping his pain at all. She was very concerned, but in a moment of frustration, snapped back, "If the shoe fits, buddy!" immediately regretting her tone and her part in upsetting poor Jim.

The truth was, Mary suspected that the pills were actually making him worse, but she couldn't get that thought through to Jim, who felt like they were his only lifeline to an otherwise miserable existence. How could she take that away from him? She had talked with the doctor about her concerns, and he assured her that Jim needed the high doses of medications in order to tolerate the intractable pain he was experiencing. He even suggested that she was out of line for expressing concern. So once again, she became the "bad guy." Her response was to clam up and withdraw from Jim even more — perhaps they were right and she was wrong. Sometimes she felt like she was going crazy. This was certainly not what she signed up for twenty-two years ago.

The Stigma of Addiction

Why are the words "addiction" and "addict" so problematic for so many people? Much of this difficulty can be attributed to the stigma that is assigned to them. *Merriam-Webster's Collegiate Dictionary* defines stigma as "a mark of shame or discredit."* It is often attached to social judgment and cultural norms. The stigma attached to "addiction" and "addict" makes them "dirty" words. Despite volumes of research on drug dependence and scientific evidence to the contrary, addiction is viewed by many as a moral failing or weakness. Addicts and their families are subjected to social, legal, and financial discrimination, making it difficult for them to obtain the help they need. When addicts do access help, insurance is inadequate to cover the cost of effective treatment. Family members are often the most judgmental because they have experienced the consequences of the addict's behavior, not realizing the addict is sick, not "bad."

Jim adamantly denied the possibility that he was an addict; after all, addicts shoot drugs, take double their prescription without permission, or get drugs on the street. Addiction is one of the few diseases that carries such a negative emotional charge and is a source of shame or embarrassment. Who would want to have a diagnosis or label that carries such a stigma? For those with chronic pain who take opioids, attempting to discuss this topic is often met with resistance and denial.

{ *exercise* 4.1 }

Your View of Addiction _____

When you hear the word "addiction" or "addict," what is your emotional response?

_____
_____
_____
_____
_____

"Addiction" is a term that often conjures up negative stereotypes. You may relate to some and not to others. Write your stereotypes about addiction. Where do these ideas come from?

_____
_____
_____
_____
_____

*By permission. From Merriam-Webster's Collegiate® Dictionary, 11th Edition, ©2008 by Merriam-Webster, Incorporated (www.Merriam-Webster.com).

Is It Really About Choice?

Many view addicts' use of substances and related behaviors as a choice. People who have addiction may have made a decision at one time to use a drug, but they never made a decision to become addicted. The addict's brain was different before the first use of a drug, and scientific evidence has shown many of the significant ways the brain changes in response to chronic exposure to mood-altering drugs. According to Alan I. Leshner, Ph.D., former director of the National Institute on Drug Abuse (NIDA), "The evidence suggests that those long-lasting brain changes are responsible for the distortions of cognitive and emotional functioning that characterize addicts, particularly the compulsion to use drugs that is the essence of addiction."

Addiction is a no-fault illness, just like chronic pain.

Even a person who never used a substance in the past and only started taking medication for his or her chronic pain may develop addiction. Just as an addict who uses for the first time is not choosing to become addicted, an individual with chronic pain who takes his or her first prescription would never choose and never intend to become addicted. For those of you who are resistant to exploring the possibility that _____ is addicted, the issue may be getting past the stigma of addiction.

It's Not Addiction Because... _____ { *exercise* 4.2 }

This exercise deals with some common misconceptions about addiction and some of the ways people deny the possibility of addiction. If you have used any of the following statements, place a check next to it. If you are undecided or don't believe _____ is an addict, write your reasons in the space below.

_____ The medications are necessary for the chronic pain.

_____ The medications are prescribed by a doctor, not illegal drugs.

_____ Addicts lie, cheat, steal, or live on skid row.

_____ Addicts snort, smoke, or inject their drugs.

_____

_____

_____

_____

_____

Problematic Drug Use (PDU)

For many with chronic pain, addiction may be too much of a stretch. You may find it helpful, however, to look at _____'s use of medications as being either problematic or nonproblematic. Even before a diagnosis of addiction is established, you may conclude there is problematic use that may or may not evolve into addiction. The following table will assist you in defining problematic use.

Table 4.1

Nonproblematic Prescription Drug Use	Problematic Prescription Drug Use
Pain is relieved or manageable with medications.	No appreciable decrease in pain.
No significant changes in functioning due to medication.	Significant decrease in functioning due to medication.
No significant effect on relationships; no concerns from family regarding use.	Ongoing relationship problems and concerns from family regarding use.
Able to work with no significant decrease in job performance.	Unable to work or significant impairment due to medication.
Stable or maintenance dose of pain medication.	Steadily increasing dose and frequency of medications with little or no decrease in pain.
Emotional stability and acceptance of any physical limitations.	Emotional instability and increasing lack of acceptance regarding physical limitations.
No significant cognitive impairment due to medication use.	Significant cognitive impairment due to use e.g., foggy thinking, difficulty concentrating, memory problems.
Using medications only for pain relief.	Relying on medications for emotional effect.

_____'s *Use of Medications*_____

Write about areas related to the table on the previous page where _____ is experiencing problems.

_____

_____

_____

_____

_____

_____

_____

If _____ is experiencing PDU, what do you believe are your options?

_____

_____

_____

_____

_____

_____

From this point on, we will use the terms "addiction" and "problematic drug use" (or "PDU") interchangeably. Use the term that feels right to you, keeping in mind that regardless of how you choose to label the situation, the principles of pain recovery apply.

How Can You Tell if Someone Has a Drug Problem?

Amy clearly met the criteria for addiction and had progressed to stage III. Jim, on the other hand, had problems as a result of his drug use, but did not clearly fall into the diagnostic category of addiction. Amy's use was driven and out of control—her search for "mood-altering effects" was clearly different from Jim's desire to reduce his pain. Jim's problematic drug use is defined by his use of the drugs to cope with life's difficulties, including pain, anxiety, fear, sleeplessness, etc.

Identifying addiction and problematic drug use in the face of chronic pain can be especially difficult for family members. How can you question a doctor's recommendations? How can you ask the person in pain to do without medication? Pain may be the driving force behind the drug-using behavior, but after awhile it doesn't matter. What matters is that the drugs have become the problem, and have actually made the pain problem worse (opioid-induced hyperalgesia). Now there is a pain problem *and* there is a drug problem (whether it is addiction or not), which is what the focus needs to be on because without treating the drug problem, there is no chance at doing anything for the rest.

Physical Signs of Problematic Drug Use and Addiction

- Increased energy, restlessness, and sleeplessness.
- Excessive sleep.
- Slow movements or reactions or abnormal speech.
- Sudden weight loss or weight gain.
- Nausea, vomiting, diarrhea, constipation.
- Fatigue.
- High or low blood pressure.
- Rapid heartbeat.
- Blood abnormalities.
- Liver abnormalities.
- Decreased libido.

Mental and Emotional Signs of Problematic Drug Use and Addiction

- Periods of being unusually cheerful, talkative, or energetic.
- Increased irritability, agitation, and anger.
- Periods of being unresponsive or looking "spaced out."
- Depression.
- Suicidal ideations.
- Anxiety.
- Hopelessness, helplessness.

- Paranoia.

- Hallucinations.

- Delusions.

Signs of Problematic Drug Use and Addiction _____

{ *exercise* 4·4 }

Describe any signs of problem drug use, from the previous lists or others you have observed, that you are concerned about in _____.

_____

_____

_____

_____

_____

On the following page you will find a self-test provided by the Pain in Recovery Support Group (PIRSG), a support group designed for people in twelve-step programs who have chronic pain and want to improve their quality of life without the use of opioid medications. You can use this exercise to assess _____'s use of medication and the possibility of addiction. You can also give copies to other family members or friends to complete. Getting input from others can help expand your view. When we are too close to a situation, those who care for us may provide perspective. If you feel resistant to doing this, just acknowledge the resistance and do it anyway. Don't prejudge what others may say; just get their input. Input is necessary to accurately assess and diagnose, and, as with any medical condition, you need an accurate assessment and diagnosis to effectively deal with your problems. So stay open-minded and get as much information about your situation as you can. If you feel the information from others is inaccurate, be sure to discuss this at a later time with a trusted person, a counselor, or a professional.

Is _____ *Addicted to Pain Medication? Checklist*

The following questions may help you make that determination. Place a check mark next to all that apply or have ever applied to _____.

_____ 1. Taking more of a medication or taking it more frequently than was prescribed.

_____ 2. Using a different doctor because a doctor wouldn't prescribe more medication.

_____ 3. Increase in the dosage of medication.

_____ 4. Looking at the clock to find out when medication can be taken next (preoccupation).

_____ 5. Using alcohol while taking prescriptions to enhance the medications' effect, even knowing it is against the directions.

_____ 6. Using illegal drugs while taking prescribed medications.

_____ 7. Having more than one doctor who is prescribing medications.

     _____ *(If checked:)* Doctors are unaware of medications being prescribed by other doctors.

_____ 8. Going to the emergency room to get additional medications because the ones prescribed were not enough.

_____ 9. Running out of a prescription too early because of using more than was prescribed.

_____ 10. Thinking "as needed" means use as much as he or she wants/needs to take.

_____ 11. Lying to a doctor about the reason for needing another prescription filled (e.g., "The dog ate my prescription," or "My pills fell in the toilet.")

Give examples of other excuses you have ever heard:

_____

_____

_____

_____

_____ 12. Exaggerating reported pain levels to get another or a stronger prescription, or "just in case."

_____ 13. Having had addiction problems before developing chronic pain.

_____ 14. Thinking, "I can't live without medication."

_____ 15. Lying to you or other family or friends about getting a prescription.

_____ 16. Lying to you or anyone about the amount of medication being taken.

_____ 17. Supplementing prescription medication with over-the-counter medication.

_____ 18. Taking other prescriptions to deal with the side effects of pain medication, e.g., sleep aids, stimulants, antianxiety drugs, or Soma.

_____ 19. Taking someone else's medication.

_____ 20. Stealing, forging, or altering a prescription.

_____ 21. Calling in a prescription by impersonating medical staff.

_____ 22. Taking medication in a way other than the way it was intended to be taken, such as crushing, snorting, or injecting it.

_____ 23. Overdosing or needing medical help as a result of taking too much medication.

_____ 24. Experiencing blackouts (memory loss) caused by medication.

_____ 25. Experiencing legal consequences as a result of taking medication, such as a DUI or assault and battery arrest.

_____ 26. Having family members, friends, or others who have expressed concern regarding medication use.

_____ 27. Taking pain medications to deal with other issues such as stress or anxiety.

_____ **How many check marks do you have?**

What are your thoughts about this?

_____

_____

_____

None of these questions necessarily defines addiction, but if you checked any of these, you should not rule out the possibility of _____ having addiction or at least problematic drug use. The more check marks you have, the greater the cause for concern about addiction.

Usually people begin taking medication to manage physical pain, but at some point, often without realizing it, start using the medication to manage emotional pain as well. Eventually the medication's effect no longer lasts as long or works as well to ease the physical or emotional pain, and the side effects may actually cause more physical and emotional pain. In the end, medication use that started as a reasonable treatment approach to relieve suffering can be the cause of problems in all areas of a person's life and place enormous strain on you, the family member.

Often those around the drug user become aware of the developing problem long before the user does, so as a family member, it is important to be alert. The user will only see that "the drugs work to take my pain away," but the big picture might come from someone who is living with him or her.

{ *exercise* 4.6 }

Pain and PDU: Four Different Stories _____

1. *JR had a history of alcohol abuse — twelve to twenty-four beers per day, shots on weekends, blackouts, and a DUI fifteen years ago. He also smoked and snorted one to two grams of cocaine per day for a few years. After his DUI, the court ordered him to attend twelve-step meetings. Much to his surprise, he attended, grew to like the meetings, got a sponsor, and worked the Twelve Steps. His recovery was going well — so well that he got married to Charlene, got promoted, and was so busy with family and work that he stopped going to meetings. Charlene, who had no experience with addiction, couldn't understand why JR had to go to "those meetings" anyway. She had never seen him drunk in the time they had been together. Six months later, he lifted a heavy box in his garage and sprained his back. An MRI showed no significant cause for his pain, and his doctor started him on Lortab and Soma, with Ambien to help him sleep. Before he realized it, he was taking the entire thirty-day prescription in the first nine days, and for the rest of the month he would beg and borrow more drugs, eventually resorting to stealing drugs from his ailing mother or buying them on the street. He would drink when he ran out of pills, which became a more frequent occurrence. Charlene was baffled by his loss of control — she had a prescription for Lortabs that lasted six months or more (until JR found it and took all the pills). She couldn't understand why he couldn't take the medications as prescribed. She wondered what was wrong with him. Clearly, JR had reactivated his addiction and required treatment, which got him re-engaged in the recovery process. He also needed to acquire tools to deal with his pain without medications. He admitted that he had been taking the pills for all sorts of reasons, including to relax, to get energy, and sometimes just to get high. Charlene needed a lot of help understanding JR's addiction and now his new attempts at recovery.*

2. *Deirdre wonders how this happened to her. She was a regular working stiff, living in a nice house with her husband Sam and two kids. She never used drugs to any great extent; she didn't like them. She had tried cocaine and pot with Sam when they were younger and got drunk on weekends in college, but that's about it. She had hardly had more than a glass of wine with dinner once a month for the past few years. She lost her taste for alcohol when she started taking pain pills. Her mom was a pill addict, and she never wanted to be like her. Then she developed pelvic pain and adhesions after surgery for endometriosis. She found that one or two Lortab in the morning took the pain away and got her going better than a double espresso. So she started using the pills to get going, keep going, and relieve the pain. When the doctor gave her Soma, she could calm down, numb out, and sleep—she was hooked. The pain was a great excuse, and her doctors were perfect accomplices. She progressed from Lortab to Percocet, which she was getting from her pain doctor, internist, GI doctor, and gynecologist, and neither she nor they realized what was happening. She eventually found that chewing the pills gave her a more intense high. A few months ago she started buying from friends, and now she is spending $500 a month on pills. She's up to twenty pills a day. Sam is furious with her—she was his high school sweetheart, love of his life, and she's turning into a stranger. Her behavior toward him and their kids is unacceptable, but he doesn't know how to make her stop. Threats fall on deaf (and stoned) ears. The fights have gotten worse and worse. His sense of powerlessness is overwhelming. Deirdre knows she is out of control, addicted, and needs help, but she's mystified—how did this happen to her? After all, it just started with the pain! She's not even sure if she's in pain or not anymore.*

3. *May wants off medications but feels she is not an addict. She never abused drugs, took anyone else's prescription, or stole to support herself. Her medications are all prescribed by her doctor. She wants to try going off meds because they have significant side effects—she is not herself. She sleeps a lot and her pain is still pretty bad. The medications don't work as well as they used to, and she's taking stronger medications in higher doses. She heard that stopping meds may decrease her pain, although she finds that hard to believe. She developed fibromyalgia ten years ago and has no life. Her husband Harry left and her grown kids don't come around, and she doesn't blame them. Harry walked out and was living with his parents. He thought that if he left, it would jolt May into changing. He was miserable, living with his folks after all these years. He was angry, frustrated, and helpless. After Harry left, May slept most of the time, and when she was awake she was depressed, grumpy, and complaining. And the constipation was killing her! She thinks of an addict as someone who lives on the street. Addicts take medications to get high. They lie, cheat, and steal. She doesn't do those things. Her dad was an alcoholic and she doesn't ever want to act the way he did. He was abusive and downright hateful. She never drank because of that, and tried pot only a few times as a kid. She takes no other drugs except what is prescribed. She doesn't buy that she's an addict and doesn't want to participate in addiction treatment, but she wants off the medications*

and doesn't know how she'll be able to live with the pain. She is consumed with fear all the time. She's angry at herself for not being stronger, at Harry for leaving, and at the doctors for allowing this to happen. Harry wants to come home, but refuses until she gets some help.

4. *Henry doesn't think he has addiction and doesn't want off his drugs, but THEY want him to stop. He sustained a fracture of his lumbar spine and herniated three discs two years previously when he fell from a scaffold at work. He hasn't worked since. He is angry at the person who left the floor wet and slippery, which caused him to slip and fall. He is furious with the worker's comp company, and especially with the case manager who wouldn't let him have another surgery and who delayed his MRI. They generally made his life miserable. He is angry at his wife for any number of reasons, and irritable with his kids. They can barely get by on the money he gets from disability, and as for his lawyer, the SOB won't even call him back. He is miserable and depressed. He is in a dead-end life that on many days he wishes would end. On Tuesday he was confronted by all of them—wife, lawyer, case manager, doctor, even his poor parents were dragged into it. He couldn't stand the tears, and in fact, he can't stand emotion at all. So he agreed to detox and try to stay off medications and do something different with his pain. On a scale of one to ten, his optimism about success was a zero, but at least he'd get them all off his back. He can't imagine living without his medications or the medical marijuana he is using. How will he sleep? he wonders (even though he never sleeps now for more than an hour or two). Medications are the only thing that made his life tolerable—that and lying perfectly still until the meds kick in and he is able to fall asleep. Not much of a life, but what else is there? He has adjusted to this life, such as it is, and now THEY want to mess it up. His wife and parents were devastated by the ultimatums they leveled—"Either get help or get out." After all, he is their "baby" and in trouble. But they reluctantly followed the advice of the doctor and went through with the intervention. Their optimism about the possibility of him getting better and giving up medications is minimal as well.*

The examples of these individuals illustrate the four types of clients seeking help for chronic pain whom we generally find in the Chronic Pain Recovery Program at Las Vegas Recovery Center:

1. Those who identify as having addiction. These are people who know they are addicts and have experienced recovery. Because of chronic pain issues, they have relapsed in an attempt to relieve or control their pain.

2. Those who had no history of addiction, but started on pain medications and now are out of control. They are addicted and unable to stop or regain control of their lives, and they are beginning to realize this and what they have to do—that is, stop the drugs.

3. Those who do not believe they are addicted. They take only medications prescribed by a doctor, *but* their lives are not better with pain-relieving drugs; in fact, their lives are worse. Even though they are taking medications, their pain is increasing rather than being controlled. Their dosages are escalating in the face of inadequate pain relief, and their function is more impaired since they have been on the drugs. They are reluctant to do anything lest it make the pain worse.

4. Those who in no way think they have a problem with their medications or addiction, but someone else thinks so. This other person may be a spouse, significant other, parent or child, employer, doctor, counselor, therapist, lawyer, judge, worker's compensation case worker, etc. Another person or organization is *making* them do something about their drug use. (Does anyone or anything really *make* someone do something?) They're in pain and they don't think it can get any better. They are convinced that coming off medication will make their pain and life worse. They may even think they need more medication, not less.

Write about which of these four types best describe your understanding of _____ and how you feel about it. These categories are not mutually exclusive. You may feel one fits best, you may relate to several, or you may not be sure which best describes _____.

_____

_____

_____

_____

_____

Write about your feelings about the families of these four types. Can you relate to any of these feelings? If so, which ones?

_____

_____

_____

_____

What You Can Do if You Suspect Addiction

If you are concerned _____ has addiction, here are some things you can do:

1. GATHER INFORMATION.

- Address your own blind spots or possible denial (in part, you have already done this by reading the material in this book on chronic pain and addiction).

- If you have trouble with this, consider going for counseling or Nar-Anon meetings.

- Talk to other family members or friends and get their viewpoint. Do they share similar concerns? Have they noticed negative changes in behavior?

- Be aware of any secrets being kept or issues being avoided by you or others.

- Go to _____'s doctor appointments and find out what the diagnosis is and any treatment it involves.

- Make a list of _____'s medications, including how long he or she has been on them, what they were prescribed for, and how they are supposed to be taken (directions).

- Notice if _____ takes the medications as directed.

- Inform yourself about _____'s chronic pain condition via the Internet or another reliable source. What are the recommended treatments for it?

2. COMMUNICATE.

- Have an honest and nonjudgmental conversation with _____ without walking on eggshells or worrying about the effect of that conversation.

- Tell _____ what you know about his or her condition and what your concerns are.

- Ask if _____ thinks there is a problem or is worried about his or her drug use.

- Talk about what you can do together to get help.

- If you can't talk about it without arguing, consider going to counseling, and be sure to go.

3. GET HELP.

☞ We encourage you to get as much support as you can in this process, including professional help. Here are some resources to use to find help and support:

- **National Institute on Drug Abuse (NIDA):** nida.nih.gov

- **Substance Abuse and Mental Health Services Administration (SAMHSA):** samhsa.gov

- **Nar-Anon Family Groups World Services:** nar-anon.org

- **Adult Children of Alcoholics (ACA):** adultchildren.org

- **Al-Anon:** alanon.org

- **Co-Dependents Anonymous (CoDA):** coda.org

- **National Family Caregivers Association (NFCA):** thefamilycaregiver.org

Finding Recovery

The process of recovery is the same whether substance use has been entirely related to a chronic pain diagnosis or it started before a person had chronic pain. Often, people with chronic pain and addiction and their families spend time and energy trying to figure out who is to blame for what has happened. We find that it is not helpful to assign blame. We want to help you stay focused on discovering and implementing solutions. In many ways, *how* your problems came to exist in your family is of minimal importance unless knowing this information helps you learn how to change your life for the better. The past is not unimportant, but you can start by knowing what the issues are in this moment and then move forward from there.

Chris finally hit the wall. He told Amy he wanted out of their relationship. That seemed to get her attention, because she became willing at that point to do something about her problem. It would also have been possible that Chris could have left the relationship and Amy could have continued in her way. But Amy depended on Chris for finances, medical care, and the like, so in essence, his leaving meant she couldn't stay as she was. Hence, his leaving precipitated a change in her. You may not have that power in the relationship you are in. You only have control over yourself, your behavior, your actions; but you can learn over time, again, with assistance, to develop some parameters around which you will tolerate and continue to participate in this relationship as it is. Our recommendation is that you set limits and stick to them, and withdraw some of what you are giving to _____ if he or she is unwilling to change behavior that is egregious.

Let's move along to pain recovery, which encompasses the solutions for bringing your life back into balance. We believe it will work for you.

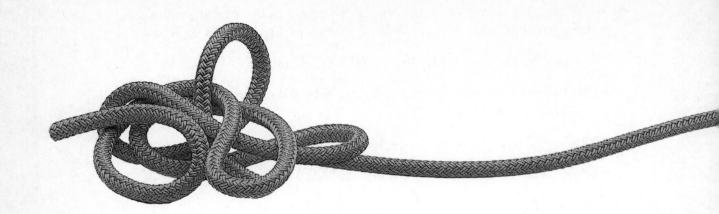

5

Pain Recovery: Finding Balance

During the months before Amy had decided to get help, Chris had just about had it with her. "What are you doing in bed? Are you crazy? You're going to get fired this time for sure!" he yelled with exasperation. He felt so powerless to help her and also to get her up and moving, but the minute he shouted and saw the tears in her eyes, he began the endless cycle of frustration, regret, sadness, and humiliation. He was frustrated that he couldn't help her, and regretful that he was stuck with such a sick person who didn't want to help herself. He felt guilty for wanting to leave and sad that he had to stay. He felt humiliated that again he shouted at her rather than being understanding. He was furious with himself and her, and he just didn't want to do it anymore.

When we wrote *Pain Recovery: How to Find Balance and Reduce Suffering from Chronic Pain*, published in 2009, we coined the term "pain recovery." The term refers to the person in pain, but in this chapter we're going to show how the exact same concepts are relevant to the family members and the family system. As we discussed in Chapter Two, the family suffers along with the person in pain and develops their own dysfunctional and imbalanced ways of thinking and behaving, often without realizing it. Over time the pain becomes the central organizing feature of the family relationship. Even as we wrote this book, we found ourselves often being drawn into the story of the person in pain; but that is not what we wanted to write about. We wanted to write about you, the person who cares about the person in pain. Nevertheless, pain is a compelling force that drives us to focus on the problem. Similar to our work in writing this book, the work of the family member is to stop spinning around the person in pain.

Amy's pain pulled and sucked Chris in, almost magnetically. Chris needed to withdraw the focus from Amy so he could stop and really look at his own life. He needed time to reflect on what he was doing, how he felt, and what his state of balance was. The first step toward finding balance is to separate from that gravitational pull of the person in pain. This might require physical separation; certainly it requires some emotional distancing. It also requires help from others, such as a skilled doctor, therapist, or somebody else who has experienced and understands what you are going through. The second step, and the focus of this chapter, is to understand the concept of balance, to discover where you are out of balance, and to work on restoring balance.

From this point forward, the work you will do in this book will be focused on establishing your own program of recovery to restore balance to your life. Obviously if the person in pain becomes healthier and more balanced, it makes your job easier. But recovery is the ability to be okay with yourself—and to not lose your sense of self—no matter what is going on around you. It requires you to develop a sense of equilibrium despite another's experience of pain. So this chapter and the chapters that follow will teach you how to be in balance despite what _____ is doing.

Pain Isn't the Whole Problem, nor Is "Curing" the Pain the Whole Solution

If a miracle occurred and suddenly _____'s pain was completely gone, everything would be fine, right? After all, isn't the pain the problem? Actually, there is more to this picture: You would still need to deal with the damage caused because of the pain. You would still have faulty thinking, and the emotional and spiritual impact of living with someone in pain for so long would remain, especially if addiction has been part of the picture. You may be in poor physical shape as a result of unhealthy eating habits, lack of exercise, and lack of adequate rest. Even though you consciously want _____ to get better, without addressing your thoughts, feelings, spirit, relationships, and behaviors, you would remain stuck, and you might not be able to tolerate the changes. You might even unknowingly sabotage recovery because you have developed an attachment to your care-giving role, which has now become your major source of identity and esteem.

As strange as it seemed to Chris, when Amy entered treatment and started working on a recovery program, stopped the drugs, and began learning to live with her pain, he found himself feeling unsettled and fearful. He had free-floating anxiety a good part of the time, especially when she was off on her own at a support group or twelve-step meeting. He found himself wondering who he was, now that Amy's need for full-time care was gone. He became confused and annoyed with himself. "After all, isn't this just what I wanted—for her to get better? And now that she's improving, I'm feeling worse."

The following exercise is designed to give you a clearer picture of the total impact of chronic pain on your life and help you to understand why "curing" _____'s physical pain alone will not solve all your problems.

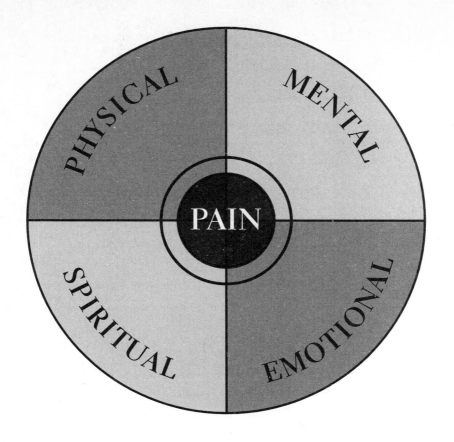

Causes of Imbalance _____

The following are issues that lead to imbalance in your life and contribute to your negative experience of having a family member in chronic pain. Check all that apply and add any that are not included.

{ exercise }
5.1

PHYSICAL IMBALANCE

_____ 1. Lack of exercise.

_____ 2. Poor eating habits.

_____ 3. Loss of physical abilities.

_____ 4. Doing too much to make up for _____'s loss of function.

_____ 5. Insomnia.

_____ 6. Sleeping too much.

_____ 7. Avoiding sex or loss of desire due to _____'s sexual problems.

_____ 8. Working excessively long hours or two jobs to support your family.

_____ 9. Other: _____

MENTAL IMBALANCE

_____ 1. Negative thoughts.

_____ 2. Thinking you are a victim.

_____ 3. Believing you have no control of your life.

_____ 4. Thinking _____'s chronic pain problem will never get better.

_____ 5. Thinking you have to do everything now that _____ has chronic pain.

_____ 6. Other: _____

EMOTIONAL IMBALANCE

_____ 1. Sad feelings.

_____ 2. Guilt and shame.

_____ 3. Anger.

_____ 4. Resentment.

_____ 5. Unresolved childhood issues.

_____ 6. Anxiety.

_____ 7. Feeling trapped.

_____ 8. Poor self-image.

_____ 9. Suicidal thoughts.

_____ 10. Other: _____

SPIRITUAL IMBALANCE

_____ 1. Anger with God.

_____ 2. Lack of trust.

_____ 3. Lack of faith.

_____ 4. Feelings of isolation.

_____ 5. Alienation from God/spirit/higher power.

_____ 6. Other: _____

Four Points of Balance for Pain Recovery

The four points of balance are applicable to any situation in life, including chronic pain in the family. The next four chapters will go into detail on each point; for now, we will give a brief overview of balance in each of the four points.

1. PHYSICAL BALANCE

Physical balance requires you to be mindful and respectful of your body, which includes paying attention to the messages it sends to your brain. You evaluate the state of your body thoroughly and continually. "How am I feeling?" "Are there any new changes in my body that I should pay attention to?" Knowing that the extra stress from having a family member in pain increases your chance of illness, you make sure to keep up on your health needs, including getting regular checkups and following the recommendations of your doctor.

With physical balance, you do things each day to take care of and strengthen your body. You understand that you cannot be a good caregiver or support for someone else if you neglect yourself.

Here are some common characteristics of a balanced physical experience:

- Eating nutritious foods.
- Exercising regularly.
- Practicing relaxation.
- Avoiding toxins.
- Getting enough sleep.
- Practicing meditation.

Patterns for Physical Balance _____

{ *exercise* 5.2 }

1. Many of our physical patterns were developed early in life. Write about some of the patterns you learned in your childhood that affect your physical balance today.

_____

_____

_____

_____

_____

_____

2. Describe your physical balance/patterns before the onset of _____'s chronic pain.

_____

_____

_____

_____

_____

_____

3. Describe how _____'s chronic pain or injury affected your physical balance/patterns.

_____

_____

_____

_____

_____

_____

4. Describe what you think will help restore your physical balance.

_____

_____

_____

_____

_____

_____

5. Describe how your relationship with _____ might be affected by restoring your physical balance.

_____

_____

_____

_____

_____

_____

2. MENTAL BALANCE

With mental balance, you challenge the assumptions and beliefs you have about _____ and his or her pain. The pain is not a punishment; it is simply an occurrence in the course of life that has various challenging ripple effects. You accept that there are some things you cannot control. Balanced thinking results in creating a realistic set of goals and focusing energy and effort into making progress toward achieving each one.

You actively and patiently change your thought patterns, knowing it happens neither easily nor quickly. However, your thoughts remain consistent in the belief that if you apply the techniques and practice the skills learned in pain recovery, your thinking will stay balanced.

You understand that having a family member in pain is stressful, and you know that you are doing the best you can. You avoid being critical of yourself during moments of frustration.

Here are some common characteristics of a balanced mental experience:

- Keeping a positive attitude.

- Paying attention to and challenging your thoughts.

- Setting achievable goals.

- Being open-minded and willing to try new things.

- Having realistic hope.

- Understanding and accepting what is real.

Patterns for Mental Balance _____

{ *exercise* 5.3 }

1. Many of our thought patterns were developed early in life. Write about some of the ways of thinking you learned in your childhood that affect your thinking today.

_____

_____

_____

_____

_____

_____

2. Describe your ways of thinking before the onset of _____'s chronic pain

_____
_____
_____
_____
_____
_____

3. Describe how _____'s chronic pain or injury affected or changed your ways of thinking.

_____
_____
_____
_____
_____
_____

4. Describe what you think will help restore your healthy thoughts.

_____
_____
_____
_____
_____
_____

5. Describe how your relationship with _____ might be affected, in a positive way, by changing the way you think.

_____
_____
_____
_____
_____
_____

3. EMOTIONAL BALANCE

With emotional balance, you accept your emotions and know that it's okay to feel whatever you are feeling. You pay closer attention to your inner voice and then take appropriate action. You are able to identify your feelings, and you recognize that your feelings are a major part of you. Noticing and accepting your feelings is therefore a major part of self-acceptance. This does not mean you wish to stay as you are, but when you first see and accept who you are in the present moment, it allows you to make positive changes in your life. Accepting your feelings takes less energy than trying to deny or suppress them. Also, accepting your feelings sometimes helps prevent them from recurring over and over and enables you to change them. Finally, fully accepting your feelings allows you to shift your energy to productive thoughts or actions.

With emotional balance you feel your full emotional experience, recognizing that all feelings are part of you—you don't need to avoid any of them. You accept your feelings without labeling them good or bad, healthy or unhealthy.

Here are some common characteristics of a balanced emotional experience:

- ☻ Understanding that feelings are neither good nor bad (not judging feelings).

- ☻ Seeing that simply experiencing emotions will not hurt you; in fact, *not* feeling emotions makes you hurt worse.

- ☻ Knowing that feeling results in healing, and avoidance results in ongoing suffering.

- ☻ Knowing that balanced thoughts create balanced emotions.

- ☻ Seeking emotional support from others.

Patterns for Emotional Balance

{ *exercise* 5.4 }

1. Many of our emotional patterns were developed early in life. Write about some of the patterns you learned in your childhood that affect how you deal with or avoid feelings today.

_____

_____

_____

_____

_____

_____

2. Describe your ways of dealing with feelings before the onset of _____'s chronic pain.

_____

_____

_____

_____

_____

_____

3. Describe how _____'s chronic pain or injury affected how you handled your feelings or how you felt toward _____.

_____

_____

_____

_____

_____

_____

4. Describe what you think will help improve how you deal with your feelings.

_____

_____

_____

_____

_____

_____

5. Describe how your relationship with _____ might be affected by changing the way you feel or handle your feelings.

_____

_____

_____

_____

_____

_____

4. SPIRITUAL BALANCE

With spiritual balance you are connected to the way you think and feel, and to how you take care of your body. When balanced, your spirituality enhances your life. You do positive things that make you feel good, and you help others. You are in harmony with the world and those in it. Whatever life brings, you are able to deal with it and know you are okay. You are able to find meaning and purpose even in situations that are painful and not to your liking. You live in and accept each day as it comes, changing yourself instead of trying to change others.

Here are some common characteristics of a balanced spiritual experience:

- Accepting who you are and your place in the world.

- Having a sense of purpose and meaning.

- Being open to challenging your beliefs.

- Drawing on a source of inner and outer strength.

- Having values, beliefs, standards, and ethics that you embrace.

- Being aware and appreciative of a "transcendent dimension" to life beyond self.

- Having increased awareness of a connection with self, others, God/Spirit/ Divine, and nature through regular spiritual practice.

Patterns for Spiritual Balance _____

{ *exercise* 5·5 }

1. Many of our spiritual patterns were developed early in life. Write about some of the patterns you learned in your childhood that affect your spirituality today.

_____

_____

_____

_____

_____

2. Describe your spirituality before the onset of _____'s chronic pain.

_____

_____

_____

_____

_____

_____

3. Describe how _____'s chronic pain or injury affected your spirituality or relationship with your higher power.

_____

_____

_____

_____

_____

_____

4. Describe what you think will help to improve your spiritual connection.

_____

_____

_____

_____

_____

_____

5. Describe how your relationship with _____ might be affected by changing your spiritual patterns.

_____

_____

_____

_____

_____

_____

Relationships

You will recognize that the more balanced you are in the four points, the better your relationships will be. Achieving this improvement will take effort on your part, and again you will find yourself changing in relationship to others.

You recognize that codependent behaviors are self-defeating both to yourself and to _____. You are able to be supportive and nurturing without being codependent or enabling. You learn healthy communication skills and apply them within the family, and you avoid isolating yourself from the world outside the family.

You ask for help whenever needed, knowing this is a sign of strength, not weakness. When you are in balance, you will attract others who have similar problems because they see the change in you and they are also interested in a solution. You freely share your solutions with them. You don't try to control them because you know everyone has to walk their own path, but you know you can provide guidance for them and share your own journey of experience, strength, and hope.

You evaluate all your relationships, looking at which ones drain you and which ones enhance your life. Knowing that drastic change will create imbalance, you create a plan to move toward building positive relationships and move away from negative relationships. You understand you will have fear, but you are aware you do not have to go through this alone.

Balanced Relationships _____

{ *exercise* 5.6 }

1. Describe how _____'s chronic pain or injury has affected your relationships within your family and with others.

_____

_____

_____

_____

_____

2. What are some things you can do to improve the quality of your relationships?

_____

_____

_____

_____

_____

Actions

As a result of continuous work to balance the four points, you are now able to face and adjust the manifestations of finding balance—your actions. Balanced actions include taking responsibility for your self-care: maintaining your health, allowing time for yourself, managing your stress, and accepting help.

You develop and execute healthy responses to troublesome thoughts and feelings. You take care of yourself by exercising, meditating, getting enough sleep, and eating properly. Right action includes the "golden rule": Do unto others as you would have them do unto you. It also includes participating in support groups and giving to others as well as receiving help.

{ *exercise* 5·7 }

Balanced Actions _____

1. What actions can you identify that are likely to change as you become more balanced?

_____

_____

_____

_____

_____

_____

The Nature of Balance

Balance is not static but fluid, in a constant state of flux much like the ebb and flow of the waves of the ocean. As the circumstances of your life change, so will your state of balance. Balance, then, is the journey, not the destination, and you are the navigator. No one else steers your ship, but people, circumstances, and events can create obstacles along the way. Like the wind, either it can blow you off course or you can harness it to move yourself in the right direction. Chronic pain is just another obstacle that you can navigate past successfully with pain recovery. Rather than viewing this as a struggle, see it as a challenge and try to find enjoyment in the journey. All that is required is that you make progress toward balance each day; there is no point of completion. Striving for perfect balance, while an admirable goal, is not a realistic one. The seas may be calm for a while, but that rarely lasts. Human beings are fallible by nature, and trying to achieve perfection would actually cause imbalance.

As you become aware of circumstances in your life that are not in balance, resist the urge to correct by oversteering. There is no quick fix, and changes are most effective when made incrementally, with all four points being considered. Imbalance often results from being unduly harsh with yourself, so resist the urge to become discouraged, to punish, or to blame yourself if you fall short of your goals. Remaining gentle with yourself is essential to establishing balance. The points represent you as a whole being, and should not be viewed as disconnected or dealt with individually without regard to each other and to the complete picture. When all four points are working in conjunction with each other, they produce a synergistic effect that is greater than each point individually.

Be aware that situations you perceive as negative and challenging, such as death of a loved one, divorce, addiction, chronic pain, getting fired, or abuse, can result in imbalance. It is important to understand that imbalance also can stem from situations you perceive as positive, such as job promotion, marriage, buying a house, or the birth of a child. Even a positive change in one point has the potential to disrupt your equilibrium. For example, if you put most of your effort into taking care of yourself physically, but don't pay attention to your thoughts, feelings, and spirit, you will be unbalanced. You might see your efforts as futile or believe they didn't work, but this is not what it means. It simply means you need to be aware that putting too much effort into one point and neglecting the others will result in overall imbalance.

The points are not a miracle cure for what ails you. Working toward balance requires diligence and persistent effort, and balancing the points can lead you to solutions for whatever you are experiencing and help you live a more meaningful and purposeful life

Balance is a dynamic mechanism that involves paying attention to yourself in the physical, mental, emotional, and spiritual areas. It gives you a path to work on and to focus on yourself, rather than being so focused on _____. The next four chapters will explore each of the four points of balance in detail and allow you to work on your state of balance in each area.

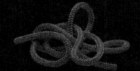

Part II

DISCOVER

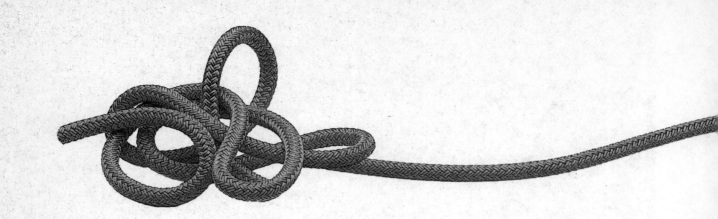

6

Physical Balance

The demands on Mary were exhausting. She slept poorly, always with an ear for Jim needing her help. He was unsteady on his feet when he awoke in the night, and fell a number of times. She felt so badly when she found him on the floor one morning, having fallen and been unable to get up. He had called for her and then dozed off in a haze from the two Ambien tablets he had taken earlier in the evening. Her only escape was to eat, and eat she did. She gained twenty-five pounds in the last year, which weighed heavily on her five-foot-four-inch frame. She had always prided herself on her fitness, exercising vigorously and often to keep in shape. Now she couldn't recall the last time she had had a good run or gone to the gym. She had to relinquish her membership a few years ago to cut back on costs.

Chris hardly slept these days. He felt depressed and hardly bothered getting up to work at his computer to facilitate sales. His job performance plummeted, and he found himself more and more frustrated with his slothful ways. He ate erratically, mostly pizza or Chinese food deliveries with occasional trips to fast food drive-thrus for carbohydrates. Ice cream became a staple in their home, since it was virtually the only thing Amy would eat. He drank more, mostly beer and wine, with a shot or two on the rare occasions he left the house to go to the corner bar. Chris found himself becoming more like Amy as the two lay around, watched TV, and dozed. At least he could be with her in this condition.

We've described the key components of finding balance in pain recovery. Now we will examine each of the four points to help you discover where you are out of balance and give you the tools to work toward restoring balance, beginning with your physical health. Most of your time and energy may be focused on _____'s physical needs because of the chronic pain, but what about your physical needs? In this chapter we will look at the physical aspects of caring for someone with chronic pain and the essential elements of good physical health. We will also describe how the brain is affected by having a loved one with chronic pain. Finally, we will present information on a number of modalities that may help improve your physical condition and that can also be done with _____ to help reduce his or her physical pain. Studies show that people in chronic pain are most helped when those closest to them encourage them to be as active as possible.

Neglecting your own physical well-being wears you down, making you unable to properly care for anyone or anything else, so don't feel guilty about making time to take care of yourself.

Physical Extremes

The most common extremes are patterns of unhealthy behaviors that cause damage to the body, including

- Inactivity (which causes joints to stiffen and muscles to weaken and atrophy resulting in a state of deconditioning).

- Overeating or eating nonnutritious foods.

- Smoking and ingesting toxic substances.

- Not sleeping enough or sleeping too much (napping throughout the day, resulting in the inability to get extended, restful sleep at night).

- Drinking alcohol excessively or taking mood-altering drugs.

Doing things that are good for you in an excessive manner is another extreme way to treat your body—for example, embarking on a vigorous course of exercise that might result in an injury or starving yourself to lose weight. Consuming alcohol or taking medications and relying on them for your well-being, to the exclusion of exercise, good nutrition, and rest, is another common example of an extreme physical behavior.

{ *exercise* 6.1 }

Inventory of Physical Imbalance _____

Write about the state of your body and your physical health now.

_____

_____

_____

_____

What behaviors or activities do you engage in regularly to maintain your physical health?

_____

_____

_____

_____

How have your physical habits changed since _____ developed chronic pain?

_____

_____

_____

_____

What physical concerns or habits do you feel you most need to address?

_____

_____

_____

_____

Therapies for Physical Balance

EXERCISE

Because of the demands of caring for _____, you may feel inclined to avoid exercise; however, exercise is one of the best things you can do to ultimately reduce your stress. Studies have shown that regular and sustained physical activity is beneficial to virtually every system in the body. During exercise your body releases chemicals called endorphins, which naturally relieve pain and tension, and also help to lessen anxiety and depression. The four major types of exercise are cardiovascular, strength training, balance, and stretching.

Some other benefits of regular exercise include:

- Helping you maintain a healthy weight.

- Increasing your energy level.

- Helping you build strength.

- Increasing serotonin level, which improves your mood and helps regulate sleep.

- Protecting and strengthening the heart and circulatory system.

- Lowering blood pressure.

- Increasing dopamine levels, which result in improved moods and increased energy.

Before beginning any exercise program, you should consult with your doctor to be sure the exercises are appropriate and helpful for your specific situation.

{ *exercise* 6.2 }

Physical Activity Level _____

What is your level of physical activity currently? List any activities that might be considered "exercise."

_____
_____
_____

What was your physical activity like before _____ developed chronic pain?

_____
_____
_____

Write some goals for exercise activities you might like to try and would be able to start, and include when you will start them.

_____
_____
_____

Foods and Nutrition

What we eat every day has a profound effect on how we feel. Our foods play a major role in our health and well-being. A healthy diet can extend our lives, help us fight many chronic diseases, lower stress, and give us a more positive outlook. And being and feeling healthy helps us feel better about ourselves.

The stress of caring for someone with chronic pain can deplete the body of certain nutrients. Eating the right foods in moderation and avoiding bad foods and toxins can restore these essential nutrients, as well relax the body and help fight anxiety and depression.

Here are some suggestions you can incorporate into your diet to help support your physical balance:

- **Don't skip meals.** Not eating regularly can contribute to or exacerbate symptoms of depression. It can also cause cravings and set you up to make bad food choices, such as sweets or unhealthy convenience foods.

- **Eat complex carbohydrates.** Whole grains, such as whole-wheat breads, cereals, pasta, and brown rice help boost serotonin levels in the brain, which promotes calmness and relaxation. Fresh fruits and vegetables are also good sources of carbohydrates and are loaded with nutrients.

- **Get enough iron and B vitamins.** Iron deficiency can cause sluggishness and inability to focus. Deficiencies in vitamin B9 (folate) and vitamin B6 have been linked to depression. Consuming enough of these important vitamins and minerals will help you cope better with stress and feel your best. Vitamin B-rich foods include bananas, nuts, potatoes, beans, and whole grains. Iron-rich foods include fortified cereals, dried fruits, broccoli, and spinach.

- **Get your omega-3s.** Foods rich in omega-3 fatty acids, such as walnuts, flaxseeds, and canola oil, have also been shown to increase serotonin production, as well as help regulate the nervous system.

- **Avoid:**

  - High-fat foods.
  - Alcohol.
  - Caffeine.
  - Sugar.

- **Learn more about good nutrition and how what you eat affects your mood, energy, and health.**

Cleaning Up Your Diet _____

{ *exercise* 6.3 }

Write about your diet in the last few weeks. What foods did you eat? If you like, create a food diary for the next week.

_____

_____

_____

_____

After compiling a list of foods, put a star next to those that are less healthy and write a plan to eliminate some of them.

_____

_____

_____

_____

SLEEP

Most people need at least seven to eight hours of restful sleep a night in order to heal, recharge, and function at their best. Mary discovered that she was less efficient at work, short-tempered with the kids, and weary most of the time. She felt compelled to sleep less so she could take care of everything and everyone. In fact, lack of sleep can drain your energy and patience, and generally make you feel awful. Depriving yourself of sleep to get everything done at your expense is not virtuous; you will be a better caretaker, spouse, parent, employee, etc., if you are well rested. If you are having trouble sleeping, be sure to talk with your doctor or get some professional help (though be careful in resorting to using medications for sleep).

REGULAR MEDICAL CARE

You may find yourself discussing _____'s condition and medical needs with a physician, but not discuss your own health. Be sure to make an appointment for yourself and other family members to get a checkup and address any health effects the chronic pain situation may be having on you.

Complementary and Alternative Medicine (CAM)

Physical balance may be found outside of conventional Western medicine. More and more Americans are trying complementary and alternative treatments for their ailments. According to a study in the *Journal of the American Medical Association*, 40 percent of Americans and more than two-thirds of the world population use complementary or alternative therapies. The quality of research supporting complementary and alternative approaches varies from therapy to therapy. As with any treatment approach, use of complementary therapies should be discussed with your doctor. These are techniques that may be helpful to _____, but you may also find them valuable in assisting you to establish your physical balance.

Acupuncture

Practitioners of acupuncture believe illness is due to imbalances of energy in the body. Acupuncture is a component of traditional Chinese medicine in which the body is seen as a balance of two opposing and inseparable forces or energy—yin and yang. Yin represents cold, slow, or passive aspects of the person, while yang represents hot, excited, or active aspects. This energy is also known as chi. Health is achieved through balancing of yin and yang, and disease is caused by an imbalance of these forces, leading to a blockage in the flow of chi.

In acupuncture, hair-thin steel needles are inserted into the body to stimulate fourteen energy-carrying channels to correct the imbalances. Acupuncture is thought to increase the release of endorphins, helping with pain and stress reduction.

Aromatherapy

Aromatherapy literally means the therapeutic use of scents to change moods. Essential oils distilled from plants, flowers, trees, bark, grasses, seeds, and fruits are used to treat a variety of ailments including fatigue, tension, stress, and pain.

Aromatherapy is also one of the fastest-growing natural remedies being used today. It works by awakening and strengthening the self-healing ability of the body. Smells can have a profound effect on our sense of well-being and body balance. The essential oils used in aromatherapy are antiseptic, antidepressant, antiviral, anti-inflammatory, detoxifying, expectorant, and analgesic.

Ayurveda

Ayurveda medical practitioners believe we're all born in a state of balance. This balance is thrown out of whack by the processes of life. These disruptions can be physical, emotional, spiritual, or combinations of all these. This is much like pain recovery. In Ayurveda, an individual's prakriti, or essential "constitution," is considered to be a unique combination of physical and psychological characteristics, as well as ways in which the body's constitution functions.

Three qualities called doshas form important characteristics of the body and control the body's activities. The doshas are called by their original Sanskrit names: vata, pitta, and kapha. Each dosha is associated with a certain body type and personality type. An imbalance in any dosha may be caused by an unhealthy lifestyle or diet, too much or too little mental and physical exertion, improper digestion, or problems with how the body eliminates waste products. A person's health will be good if he or she returns to balance and has a wholesome interaction with the environment.

According to Ayurveda, a person's chances of developing certain types of diseases are related to the way doshas are balanced, the state of the physical body, and mental or lifestyle factors.

Biofeedback

Biofeedback is a technique that can help you learn to control some normally involuntary processes by raising your awareness of signals from your body. This is accomplished using specialized equipment that allows you to monitor bodily functions such as blood pressure, heart rate, muscle tension, sweat gland activity, and skin temperature. In general, those who benefit most from biofeedback have conditions that are brought on or made worse by stress.

Meditation

One specific meditative practice is called the body scan, which is adapted from an ancient Burmese practice. Jon Kabat-Zinn, Ph.D., writes in *Full Catastrophe Living* that the body scan "is an effective technique for developing both concentration and flexibility of attention simultaneously. It involves lying on your back and moving your mind through the different regions of your body." This guided meditation encourages you to scan through your body much like a CT scan machine might. One key is to simply notice the sensation without judging it. It utilizes the breath to affect and decrease tension and pain. Each time you encounter these feelings you can replace them with a sense of spaciousness, relaxation, and freedom.

Chi Kung (Qigong)

Chi Kung, also known as Qigong, is a Chinese practice that integrates physical postures, breathing exercises, and mental focus. The word "Chi" means life force or vital energy, and "Kung" means skill achieved through consistent practice. Practitioners of Chi Kung believe most physical problems, including pain and diseases, are related to imbalances of vital energy fields, and that by restoring your internal/external balance you can maintain health and promote healing and vitality. Research has confirmed many of the benefits of the practice.

Chi Kung is moving meditation, and is a very gentle form of exercise that can be practiced by all age groups and can be easily modified for those with physical challenges. Specific exercises help release negative energy and focus on specific areas of the body, such as the spine. With consistent practice, Chi Kung can help you develop a more positive outlook, restore balance, and enhance quality of life.

Chiropractic

Chiropractic therapy diagnoses and treats problems involving nerves, bones, muscles, and joints. Chiropractors believe that manipulation of muscles, the spine, and other joints helps the body heal itself. Chiropractic medicine is the third largest health profession in the Western world. More than 20 million people are treated each year.

Manipulation is the primary treatment offered by chiropractors, although there are other therapies offered including massage and prescribed exercises. Chiropractors sometimes use various tests to help with their diagnoses such as X rays, blood tests, and blood pressure readings.

Although chiropractic medicine has a lot in common with other health professions, it is unique in its belief that spinal misalignment is the cause of most forms of illness. Many people visit a chiropractor for a specific problem; however, chiropractors report that their manipulations benefit the person's health in a general way. There are hundreds of different techniques and methods of manipulation used by chiropractors to treat as many conditions. Research has shown that chiropractic medicine is effective in many cases to reduce and treat acute and chronic back pain. It also has been shown to help many painful conditions including frozen shoulder, muscle spasms, and carpal tunnel syndrome, among others.

Hypnotherapy

Hypnotherapy uses concentration, relaxation, and focused attention to attain a heightened state of awareness called a trance or hypnotic state. The person in the trance becomes able to block out outside stimuli and concentrate on specific tasks or thoughts. It is used to help people perceive stimuli differently, such as by blocking the perception of pain. Hypnotherapy can be used to produce deep relaxation to lower fear, tension, and anxiety.

Hydrotherapy/Hydro Massage

Hydrotherapy involves the therapeutic use of water to maintain health and to treat and prevent disease. According to proponents, there is no medicine on the market that can rival the beneficial physiological effects of water. Maintaining hydration is necessary for the function of all vital organs. Benefits of hydrotherapy include helping with sleep, controlling temperature, providing derivative pain relief, and acting as an anticonvulsant. Hydro massage is a popular treatment that uses water to apply massage techniques. This therapy can relieve muscle pain and tension, improve circulation, promote relaxation, and reduce stress and anxiety.

Massage

As a treatment, massage is used in conventional medicine as well as in CAM. The basic goal of the massage therapist is to increase the flow of blood and oxygen to a specific area of the body, relax and warm the soft tissues, and decrease pain by pressing, rubbing, and moving soft muscles and other tissues, primarily using the hands and fingers.

People use massage for any number of reasons and health-related purposes including for general wellness, for rehabilitation, to increase relaxation, to decrease stress, to help alleviate feelings of depression or anxiety, and to relieve pain. There is no doubt that a soothing massage can ease the pain of a long day and soothe achy joints and muscles.

Music Therapy

Music therapy is the clinical use of music to treat patients with physical, psychological, cognitive, and social functioning issues. It is a powerful and noninvasive method to reduce pain, anxiety, and depression. The treatment is for patients of all ages, with outcomes based on the individual's emotional, cognitive, and interpersonal responsiveness to the music and/or therapy relationship.

As a form of sensory stimulation, music provokes responses based on familiarity, predictability, and feelings of security. Therapists use musical activities, both instrumental and vocal, to cause changes in a patient's condition. Music treatment has been used to reduce stress and anxiety, help patients manage pain without drugs, and encourage positive changes in mood and emotional states.

Reflexology

Reflexology promotes healing through stimulation of points in the hands and feet, which are divided into zones that correspond to parts of the body. This natural therapy is said to help identify blockages, reduce stress and tension, promote healing and relaxation, improve circulation, eliminate toxins, and restore equilibrium. The treatment is not painful, and most people find it relaxing. Reflexology can be beneficial for many conditions and for improving general health and well-being.

Reiki

Reiki promotes good health through relaxation, stress relief, and pain management. In reiki, "universal life-force energy" is transmitted through the hands of a therapist from the vast pool of energy that abounds in the universe. Also called "palm healing" and "energy medicine," reiki is made up of two Japanese words: "rei," meaning universal spirit or spiritual wisdom, and "ki," meaning energy or life-force energy.

In CAM, energy therapies are based on the assumption that illness and pain are caused by disturbances in a person's energy. Reiki practitioners seek to improve the flow and balance of positive energy and reduce negative energy in a way that is beneficial to clients. The energy flows wherever it is needed and often is reported as a tingling in the body. Most report being extremely relaxed after a reiki treatment.

Reiki treatments have been used to reduce chronic pain, help with recovery from anesthesia and surgery, improve immunity, improve mental clarity, and lower a person's heart rate. Reiki practitioners often report clients experiencing a "cleansing crisis" after a session, in which they have feelings of nausea, tiredness, or weakness because of the release of energy toxins.

Yoga

Yoga is a Sanskrit word meaning "union." It can be thought of as a form of exercise developed over thousands of years in India. It promotes health and happiness by working on the mind, body, and spirit. Yoga is being used more and more as a treatment modality. Where the techniques and benefits of yoga were once in doubt as a therapy, physicians are now turning to it as a viable treatment for many different conditions, including pain.

Yoga works on stretching and strengthening the body. By increasing strength, improving flexibility, and ridding the body of muscle tension, a person can bring their body into balance. Practicing yoga can allow someone to focus on positive aspects of life. Deep breathing has physical and psychological benefits that can help calm the extreme emotional effects of, for example, living with chronic pain. There are now hundreds, if not thousands, of different "styles" of yoga, each promoting a different path to similar conclusions.

As Mary began to enter her own form of pain recovery, she restarted her yoga class, which had always been a source of peace and exercise. After a few weeks, she started to feel the "juices flowing" again. She rested better and felt more energetic during the day. And she worked an extra shift monthly so she could afford the luxury of a massage and spa day.

Improving Physical Balance _____

{ *exercise* 6.4 }

Write a list of complementary and alternative approaches you have tried. Be specific and include the effects you noticed and which have been helpful for you.

_____

_____

_____

_____

_____

Which ones might be helpful for you to try or resume?

_____

_____

_____

_____

What barriers might come up to keep you from following through with these plans?

_____

_____

_____

_____

Write three ways you could get assistance so you can follow through with these plans.

_____

_____

_____

_____

Now that you have begun to look at your physical state, hopefully you can see how to move in the direction of physical balance. Chances are, as you make changes, you will find that you have thoughts and emotions about changing. We will discuss these processes of the mind in the following two chapters.

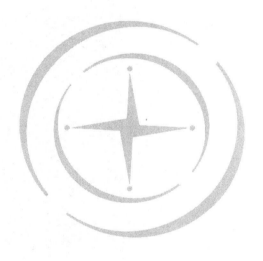

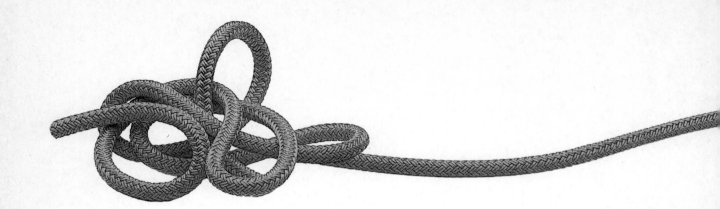

7

Mental Balance

Before Jim's injury, life was good. Like most people, Jim and Mary had plans, hopes, and dreams for their future. With the good job and income that Jim had, they talked for hours about vacations they would like to take, improvements they could make to their home, and making sure they could afford college for the kids, especially Mandi, who'd consistently gotten top marks in school. And Mary knew in her heart that Jim would always take care of his family and her, that she could count on him in that respect. She enjoyed watching Jim play with their son Ross, and remembers thinking how he was every bit the man she had fallen in love with way back when. But then Jim hurt his back, and with the pain becoming chronic, all of those hopes, dreams, and plans now seemed to be vanishing into thin air. "How could this be happening to US?" she would wonder aloud. "Why can't he just get better already?" Mary even noticed that her respect for Jim had lessened as she watched her husband struggling to get around, getting irritable and moody with her and the kids. She found herself thinking, "This isn't the man I married," and even wanted to tell him to "get over it," even though she knew in her heart that he could not just do that. As she watched her kids with their dad, she could see them losing respect for him, making sarcastic remarks or turning to her for help with the things he used to do with them. Mary and the kids were doing more and more things without Jim, and the kids would even talk about how he never wanted to do anything with them anymore. Ross even asked, "Why is Dad mad at me?" Mary could feel her family being torn apart by the strain and wanted to make it stop. She worried that it would never end.

Chris couldn't shut his mind off. He conjured up all sorts of scenarios. When he was with Amy, the stories he told himself centered on what a dope he was to put up with her. He imagined what other people thought of him, including his mom who had died years ago. He heard his mother's voice telling him that Amy was no good and he should get out now, that waiting would only make it harder. Even though she had an occasional lucid hour, or even, on occasion, a few good days, his mind told him it was going to get worse and there was no way out. He tried to blot out the thoughts with alcohol, but he simply ended up with a hangover and no further along to finding a solution. He had never come up against such a seemingly unsolvable problem.

Imbalance in thinking consists of misguided assumptions, distorted thoughts, and faulty conclusions in family members that form the basis for their reactions to the person with chronic pain. Your reactions, along with _____'s reactions and his or her thoughts, help to create imbalance in the family system, contributing to both distance between members and increased tension within the family. This increased tension may be experienced by _____ as increased pain, and you might experience the "pain" of distancing, strain, and isolation. Your perceptions are also important, especially as they pertain to _____ and the effects of that condition on your family.

Think That You Are Your Thoughts? Think Again.

When you look at the word "thought" or "think," what comes to mind? There's the first clue—we conceptualize a thought in our mind. In this chapter we will explore the point of balance most directly related to our minds and the net product of our minds' work—our thoughts. Your thoughts have a powerful influence on the way pain is experienced by _____ and on how you respond to him or her. And how you respond to pain can greatly affect balance in your family, promoting recovery or hindering it.

Unchallenged, unhealthy thoughts create a burden
too heavy for you to carry.

According to *Merriam-Webster's Collegiate Dictionary*, thought is "reasoning power; the power to imagine; a developed intention or plan; or the intellectual product or the organized views and principles."* Thoughts and thinking are based on considering information that we come in contact with, analyzing this information, and forming conclusions as to what it means. Where do our thoughts come from? How are they formed and changed? Before we discuss the mechanics of thought, we will present extremes of thought common to people who care for someone with chronic pain, and which also apply to addiction. Extreme thinking significantly contributes to an overall lack of balance in our lives.

*By permission. From Merriam-Webster's Collegiate® *Dictionary, 11th Edition, ©2008 by Merriam-Webster, Incorporated (www.Merriam-Webster.com).*

Extremes of Thinking

As pain becomes chronic, family members tend to start to view the quality of their own lives in terms of whether the pain patient is better or worse, and lose the ability to separate their sense of self from the daily function of caring for someone with chronic pain. One extreme of thinking is defining yourself by how the person in pain is doing. The belief becomes "If _____ had a good day, then I was good today; if _____ had a bad day, then I was bad today."

Another good example of this is when Jim refused to come on family outings because of increased pain, Ross would often wonder if his father was mad at him or, worse, didn't love him.

Basing your well-being on _____'s well-being can also lead to extreme thought processes rooted in fear and negativity, such as fear that he or she will get worse or become disabled, or will never be able to go back to work. You may have drawn the same faulty conclusions as Chris had, such as "This is the way it will always be," and "I don't want to live this way; my life is over." Chronically negative thinking actually makes "bad" situations worse. You may ruminate (go over and over a situation in your mind, replaying it unproductively) or magnify the negative, exaggerating the significance of something that occurred and turning what was really only a small problem into a major disaster in your mind. By focusing on the negative aspects of your experience, you actually make your life more negative. Your thoughts have the capacity to make you miserable. Negative thinking can be especially insidious, feeding on itself, with the potential to become a self-fulfilling prophecy. Because the effects of chronic pain on the family are generally so unpleasant, it is relatively easy for you to become trapped in a web of negativity from which it can be difficult to escape.

On the other side of this spectrum is to virtually "skip over" thoughts entirely (think too little), and to believe that everything is fine no matter what—refusing to acknowledge how terrible the situation really is. This can be mislabeled as positive thinking, but it's really a potentially dangerous way of thinking that flies in the face of reality, commonly referred to as denial. In this case, the pendulum swings to the extreme of not seeing reality as it truly is. This can lead to consequences such as underestimating potential problems, not taking care of yourself, and ignoring negative realities. For example, you truly don't see the nature of the drug problem that has developed. Mary and Jim's daughter was like this. In fact, when Mary tried to sit and have a conversation with her about Jim's drug use and decreased function, she refused to talk, instead saying, "Everything is fine; you're such a drama queen. Just leave me out of your issues with Dad!" and storming out of the house.

Another extreme is to view the situation in absolutes—the person in pain is either cured or not cured—rather than as a process of improving or getting better. The belief that well-being has to be pain-free may result in extreme thinking toward the person in pain along the lines of "I will do anything to keep _____ out of pain." This may lead to sacrificing your own life just to focus on keeping him or her free from pain. Or you may encourage _____ to "take a pill" whenever he or she complains of pain, thereby enabling him or her to take drugs abusively.

Your thinking may or may not take you to these extremes, but having a family member with chronic pain or addiction or both typically includes experiencing various degrees of distorted, out-of-balance thinking. Imbalance in thinking can cause imbalances in emotional, physical, and spiritual functioning.

Thinking About Thinking

Have you ever considered why you think what you think? Does it seem like your thoughts are who you are? The reality is that nothing could be further from the truth. Your thoughts are part of you, but only a part of the much greater whole. Descartes, a famous philosopher, said, "I think, therefore I am." This statement represented a step forward in the evolution of Western philosophy. However, in suggesting there is no separation between people and their thoughts, it has also has done a disservice to our understanding of the relationship between our thoughts and who we *are*. Because they occur so automatically and seem so natural, we may become so closely identified with our thoughts that we believe there is no separation: Our thoughts are us and we are our thoughts. And yet, the reality is that thoughts are mental products generated in our brain.

We also tend to believe in the inherent truth or accuracy of our thoughts, believing "I think it, therefore it is true." Assuming our thoughts are facts—that they are all true and valid without examination—is one of the reasons we find ourselves out of balance.

Chris finally talked to his brother who ironically had also been married to an addict. His message came through loud and clear: "All addicts lie, cheat, and steal. Like my ex, Amy will eventually break your heart and your bankbook." The more he heard his brother's words, the more true they seemed. Despite his waning desire to see Amy get help, the words "leave her" echoed in his brain like a mantra. As long as he thought it would never get better, it was hard to find reasons to stay, yet he was still there.

Before emotion or action takes place in any situation, a thought process occurs; but it can happen so quickly and automatically that you're not consciously aware of it. These seemingly natural, automatic thoughts are also known as "self-talk"—the things you tell yourself about what is occurring that also define your beliefs about those events. While you may be powerless over the self-talk that first enters your mind, you are not powerless over what you do in response to it. You can detach from your thoughts—observe them, question their accuracy, dispute or talk back to them, and, ultimately, change them.

Self-Talk _____

Identify your automatic thoughts or self-talk about _____'s chronic pain.
{examples:"The man I married wouldn't let pain stop him like that," or "She couldn't be hurting *that* much."}

_____

_____

_____

_____

_____

_____

Now examine each thought and describe if it is true or not.

_____

_____

_____

_____

_____

_____

What things have you done as a result of your thoughts that have increased conflict or distance within the family?

_____

_____

_____

_____

_____

_____

Pain recovery teaches that we are not what we think. We can observe our thoughts and we can dispute them by not buying everything they are trying to sell us. Paying attention to your thought process and consciously questioning and challenging your thinking is an indication of mental balance. The more consciously aware of this process you can become, the more you will be able to develop the capacity to intentionally adjust your thinking and self-talk to cope with the effects of _____'s pain more effectively.

Progress toward healing and balance also requires accepting that you cannot control your thoughts, but you can *modify* and *redirect* them. This requires the willingness to surrender, and the action of challenging and redirecting your thoughts in order to achieve balance. Learning to view and respond to your thoughts differently will require going through a process of adjustment, but by becoming more aware of and modifying your thoughts, you can improve negative effects on the family as a whole and your relationship with _____.

Not everything you think is necessarily true or accurate.

{ *exercise* 7.2 }

Thought Patterns _____

Write about a pattern of thinking you have developed that is not helpful to you but that you do not want to change.

_____
_____
_____
_____
_____

Why do you insist on holding onto those thoughts?

_____
_____
_____
_____
_____

How can you change them to be more helpful?

_____
_____
_____
_____
_____

How Self-Defeating Thoughts Create Imbalance

Imbalances of thought, wherein our minds approach what is happening in our external reality in an inaccurate way, are a common phenomenon. Our minds have the responsibility and challenge of making sense of our experience in the world so that we can understand it. Depending on external circumstances and internal influences, the mind can easily make errors in interpreting our experiences, thus throwing us out of balance.

To better understand how _____ thinks, it is important to be aware that the mechanics of thinking can be significantly distorted by pain and pain medications. Pain can take up so much space in a person's thinking that little room is left for the healthy consideration of available options. Opioid pain medications can dull and cloud the thought process, making imbalanced thinking, twisted beliefs, and inaccurate interpretations of events and situations much more likely. Family members also fall prey to these kinds of distortions, either in reaction to those of the person with pain or due to other reasons such as their past experiences with pain and illness, or their own inner turmoil.

The following sections focus on some specific and common imbalances in thinking that may be contributing to your suffering. These self-defeating thoughts have the potential to sabotage your efforts to achieve balance in the family. We will describe these patterns in some detail, have you look at how each might affect your pain and your life, and then offer solutions congruent with pain recovery.

Self-Esteem/Self-Image

_____ may have become so identified with his or her pain that it becomes part of his or her core identity. The attention, concern, and sympathy received from the family, medical professionals, and significant others serve to reinforce this self-perception and identification as a sufferer and/or victim. Many people who live with chronic pain can, over time, come to define their sense of self in terms of their pain and impaired functioning. "I used to be able to do this or that" or "I used to provide better for my family" have roots in reality for some, but can also equate to "I am very weak" or "I'm no longer valuable to my loved ones." And you may find that your identity has now become _____'s partner, spouse, child, or parent. You are now defining yourself by your role with _____ and his or her pain.

While Jim and Mary still talked, their discussions always seemed to be about the pain—what to do about it, and inevitably about all of the things Jim could no longer do because of it. There seemed to be no solutions, just an endless and hopeless discussion that left both of them feeling frustrated, angry, and depressed. As time went on they seemed to talk less and less, because neither one of them wanted to talk about that hopeless topic again! Mary became Jim's caregiver, nursemaid, and money-earner instead of the wife and mother roles she had cherished before he got hurt.

Maintaining a balanced sense of self is essential to overall health. As a family member, you are in a unique position to give _____ a perspective on his or her true value to you and the family. Thus, you can provide an important alternative perspective role to counterbalance the skewed one that has been a consequence of chronic pain. Family members will also benefit from the more balanced perspective described above, as _____ will likely become less isolated from the family.

Just as _____'s self-image and self-talk can become increasingly negative, focused on the things he or she is no longer able to do, so too can the family's focus become much more negative. The focus of family members may be more on the extra burden of work, all of the activities they no longer are able to engage in, or their perceived ineffectiveness at being unable to cure the pain. As this happens, your self-image and self-talk can become increasingly negative and focus nearly exclusively on your losses and deficits. This may happen gradually enough that you are unaware of the changes in your thinking and the way you view yourself. It is not unusual to be defensive about this and be unwilling or unable to admit to yourself and others how badly you are feeling about yourself. You may overcompensate by trying to be perfect at the things you can do. Or, since having a "normal life" together may now seem impossible, family members may withdraw from one another, leading increasingly isolated, lonely, or parallel lives. The pain recovery process encourages all members of the family to look specifically at what they think and feel about both themselves and other members of the family—particularly about the person with pain. Abilities, limits, and what really matters to you are all important. This is part of the process of change that will lead you back to balance and the life you want to live.

{ *exercise* 7·3 }

Improving Self-Image _____

Describe your self-image. What changes can you make in your thoughts to improve your self-esteem?

_____

_____

_____

_____

_____

How was your self-image affected by the onset of _____'s chronic pain/injury?

_____

_____

_____

_____

_____

Describe _____'s self-image. How does your image of _____ differ from his or her self-image?

_____

_____

_____

_____

_____

Describe how your image of _____ was affected by the onset of chronic pain.

_____

_____

_____

_____

_____

Noticing Your Thoughts

Pain recovery includes working on consciously structuring your thought process to allow for acknowledgment and recognition of your thoughts without overreacting to them. Slowing down the thought process is the beginning of this process and will help you move toward balance. Instead of identifying your thoughts as indisputable facts, allow yourself to observe them with interest and curiosity. With practice, you will be able to witness your thoughts as they arise in your awareness.

Chris had a sort of epiphany one day when he finally, out of desperation, found himself opening up to a supportive friend about his plight. His friend pointed out some facts: Amy was not Chris's ex-sister-in-law, and it was not inevitable that they split. Amy was the love of his life. Chris's thoughts had turned her into someone she wasn't—bad, selfish, cold. As he noticed and began to challenge these automatic thoughts, he found that he was able to remember how much he loved Amy. He saw that she was suffering, both with her pain and with her addiction. She was neither selfish nor bad. This freed him to reinvest in the relationship and plan an intervention to help Amy see the truth.

{ *exercise* 7·4 } ### *Slowing and Observing Thoughts* _____

Take a few moments and observe your thoughts as they come up for you right now. Write three that come to mind.

_____

_____

_____

_____

_____

Take a little time each day to practice these strategies to observe your thoughts and slow them down. We suggest you write about this daily in a separate journal or notebook.

Discounting the Positive

As we've discussed, the sheer discomfort of chronic pain often results in negative thought patterns for everyone in the family. One form these thoughts can take is to ignore, dismiss, or otherwise not be aware of anything remotely positive about this situation, whatever it may be. You and other family members may tend to focus exclusively on what _____ can no longer do or the costs of medical care or the loss of income. With or without your knowledge, you end up focusing all your conscious attention and energy on the negative aspects of the situation. For example, you hear from ten people how well you seem to be doing, while a single person tells you, for whatever reason, that you don't seem to be doing well. Rather than believe the ten people with positive views, you are certain that the one negative perspective is correct. In addition to feeding your negativity, this can also serve the self-defeating purpose of confirming what you believe about yourself—that you are not doing well. We find evidence in real events to support the position we've already taken.

In order to counteract this and reestablish balanced thinking, it is essential to keep in mind that nearly all situations and events have both positive and negative characteristics. Sometimes you may have to look a little harder or even do some work to locate the positive, but if you search for it, you will find it. Something else you can do to counteract this form of thinking is to identify things or people you are grateful for. Practicing expressing gratitude can improve mood and measurably increase the experience of happiness.

Mary became convinced that she had made a mistake marrying Jim. She focused on all his flaws and became more and more unhappy. However, the truth was that she didn't want to leave him. When she allowed herself to see Jim as he had been before the injury—a warm, loving, solid, supportive partner—she realized that he still had all those traits that had become obscured by the pain they both lived with.

Seeing the Positive

{ *exercise* 7.5 }

Describe the negative aspects of _____'s pain. Describe how these negative aspects affect your life.

_____

_____

_____

_____

_____

Now take a closer look and identify some positive aspects about it.

_____

_____

_____

_____

_____

Identify things or people that you are grateful for and briefly describe the reason(s) for your gratitude.

_____

_____

_____

_____

_____

Identify things about _____ that you are grateful for, and briefly describe the reason(s) for your gratitude.

_____

_____

_____

_____

_____

Making Mountains Out of Molehills

Some of us have a tendency to get caught up in spinning elaborate scenarios related to events that may never actually occur, and spend considerable time and emotional energy looking for potential trouble, as well as for solutions to problems that don't exist. When pain becomes chronic, the fact that it is always there can lend itself to this process. Fantasizing, after all, can be about positive and pleasurable things or negative and disastrous possibilities. For instance, when Amy rejected Chris's sexual advances, saying she was not in the mood because of pain, Chris's self-talk told him, "This is horrible! What's the use? Our sex life will never be the same. Why do I even try?" Rather, he could remind himself that pain has its ups and downs and that she will likely be more interested later on.

Thinking that catastrophe is upon you has considerable influence on your reactions to _____'s chronic pain, your relationship with him or her, and your perceived options.

The first step in interrupting this process is to become aware of it and realize what you are thinking. Only then can you make an informed decision about how you want and need to proceed based on the options available.

{ *exercise* }
7.6

Keeping Things in Perspective _____

Describe a situation where your thinking about _____'s pain caused you to make things worse for yourself, for both of you, or for your relationship.

_____

_____

_____

_____

_____

Describe how you can think differently in order to regain balance (be as specific as you can).

_____

_____

_____

_____

_____

"Black-and-White" Thinking

Thinking in "either/or" terms, where things are the complete opposite of one another with nothing in between, creates imbalance in thinking by viewing events, situations, and people (including yourself) in one of only two mutually exclusive ways: all good or all bad. Everything is either "great" or it's "horrible." The family member with pain is either in constant pain or must be totally pain-free. Self-perception tends to be based on the extremes of "I am perfect"/"I am a total failure."

Chris's thinking was along the lines of "I can't get out. I have to stay with Amy no matter what because she is sick." He believed he had no other options. Mary took on a nurselike role for Jim and believed she had to care for all the needs of the family at the expense her own needs and desires. Overburdened and unable to see any solutions, she spiraled into depression and began self-medicating with food.

Your thinking may shift from one extreme to the other, depending on circumstances. In this thought pattern there is no middle ground. In fact, most of reality occurs somewhere in the middle, between the black and white and within those many shades of gray, not to mention the endless palette of colors that enrich our everyday experiences. When you are unable to see and appreciate this middle ground, you end up missing much of the richness and subtlety of life.

You can regain balance by becoming consciously aware of this tendency, checking your thought process, and noticing when you are thinking in black-and-white terms. This awareness will provide the opportunity to look for the middle ground—the shades of gray that you are missing.

*Seeing the Shades of Gray*_____

Describe examples of when you have engaged in black-and-white thinking. Use the prompts provided or list other examples.

Success vs. Failure:

_____

Sick vs. Well:

_____

Happy vs. Sad:

_____

Good vs. Bad:

_____

Other:

_____

_____

_____

_____

_____

Now, identify the shades of gray that exist between the two extremes.

_____

_____

_____

_____

Expectations of Yourself and Others

Everyone has beliefs about how things *should* be in relation to themselves, to others, and to the world. Expectations usually involve judging yourself, others, and situations against specific standards for behavior and reality that you've created in your mind.

Sometimes these expectations become imperatives, such as "Things *must* be the way I want them to be." Whenever you think in terms of how people or situations should be, you set yourself up for disappointment. For example, maybe you expected that _____'s pain condition would improve after that last surgery or procedure, or that he or she was going to be back to work by now. These beliefs and expectations come from past influences and a lifetime of experiences. If one of your parents or siblings got sick or injured, how did your family react to them? Did they allow them to be sick for a time or expect them to act as if nothing happened? We all learned about how long you are allowed or expected to be sick. From this we often get our ideas or expectations about how long sickness will last and when to start wondering of something else is wrong.

When you don't perform as you think you should; when others don't act as you think they should; when situations don't turn out as you think they should, the resulting emotions are likely to include guilt, shame, frustration, hurt, and anger. For people and their families struggling with chronic pain, this can create serious imbalances in both thinking *and* emotions. Mary would often find herself having thoughts such as "It's not fair that Jim got hurt and now can't work. We should still be able to do all the things that we used to do. This shouldn't have happened, and he should not have to live with the pain."

A solution to restore balanced thinking when you're caught up in expectations is to consciously separate what you may want from the reality of the situation. It's normal, natural, and understandable to want things the way you want them. But mental balance and pain recovery require you to develop the ability to accept the things you cannot change. Applying the Serenity Prayer (see below) and identifying the things you cannot change, as well as what you can do to better accept those things, will make noticeable, positive differences in your experience of pain and in your life. It is essential to remember that one thing you can always change is how you respond to the people, events, and situations in your life.

Applying the Serenity Prayer _____ { *exercise* } 7.8

Grant me the serenity to accept the things I cannot change, courage to change the things I can, and wisdom to know the difference.

Identify something about _____'s chronic pain or its effect on your family that you cannot change and need to accept.

_____

_____

_____

_____

Describe how you will begin to go about accepting it.

_____

_____

_____

_____

Identify something about _____'s chronic pain or its effect on your family that you can change.

_____

_____

_____

_____

Describe how you will begin to go about changing it.

_____

_____

_____

_____

Describe how you can tell the difference between what you can and cannot change.

_____

_____

_____

_____

Family members can also have unrealistic expectations of themselves and of other family members, believing that they can carry too much of the burden. They may view it as selfish to take care of themselves, when in fact the opposite is true. Studies have shown that people who provide care for a family member with chronic illness are less likely to attend to their own health care needs, less likely to eat properly and exercise, and more likely to abuse alcohol. Studies have also found that caregivers are at increased risk of developing a chronic disease themselves. This is why it is necessary for you to take care of yourself and to work on your own state of balance, because by forgetting your own well-being you may get sick and become unable to take care of anybody.

Applying Your Knowledge of Thoughts _____

Here are some examples of family members' thoughts about the people in their families who have chronic pain. From the chapter you've just completed, see if you can figure out what type of thinking is reflected in these examples.

THOUGHT	TYPE OF THINKING
"Why won't she try harder? She won't even try to do better."	
"I just want our life to be normal again."	
"His pain will never go away."	
"We'll never have a normal life together again."	
"She couldn't be in that much pain. Doesn't she want to work?"	
"I've lost my husband."	
"She isn't the woman I married anymore."	
"Our sex/love life is over."	
"I have to avoid talking about or doing certain things because he can't do them anymore because of his chronic pain"	
"My mother doesn't love/care about me anymore because she can't play with me or do the same things or is always mad at me."	
"When he gets all better, then we can have fun again."	
"Things would be better if he'd only try harder."	
"Why doesn't she want/love me anymore?"	
"He is so weak."	
"Maybe if I tried harder and did more for him, things would be better."	
"Maybe if I did more or acted differently…"	
"Maybe if I was stronger…"	
"I can't be emotional or weak—I have to be strong and logical."	
"If I just keep helping her look for the right doctor/medicine/procedure, everything will be fine."	

At this point in your recovery process, you have learned about your body and how the mind, specifically your thinking, is a powerful force in affecting your state of balance. The next chapter will introduce the concept of emotional balance and the importance of emotions on your well-being.

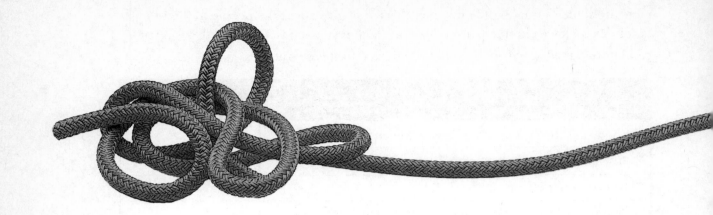

8

Emotional Balance

Mary rarely had a moment to herself between work, Jim's doctor appointments, pharmacy runs, and waiting on him when she was home. She felt ashamed that she wished she could just run away and leave this burdensome life behind. She was miserable and angry and frustrated and fearful about the future. She didn't feel she could talk to anyone about these feelings; after all, "What kind of a wife resents her husband who is in pain?" she would ask herself when she found herself driving the long way home to prolong the few minutes she had without responsibility. The worst part of it for Mary was to watch Jim when he was in pain. She felt so helpless and powerless, seeing the man she loved experiencing discomfort. It was as if she was feeling the pain herself sometimes. Her heart would break, and sometimes she even wished it were her who had been in the accident and was suffering—that seemed better than the powerless feeling of watching his distress.

Chris's default emotion became anger. He was angry at Amy for the things she did, at himself for being inconsiderate and impatient, at their friends for "disappearing" when he really needed them. He lived angry, slept angry, and awoke chronically in a bad mood, and he was sick of it.

As we discussed in the previous chapter, the mind and body share such intimate connections that they affect each other in direct and powerful ways. Emotions are part of the circuitry that links mind and body. Having a close relationship with someone in chronic pain causes a multitude of difficult emotions. Even when feelings are uncomfortable or painful, they are sending us important messages that can help us make sense of what is happening. Finding emotional balance does not mean you will not experience difficult feelings or go through hard times. It means developing your ability to recognize your emotions and express them appropriately, as well as having a sense of emotional connection with others and a strong support system. Thus, with emotional balance you are able to cope with stressful situations and life's inevitable challenges and still remain productive and positive.

A common characteristic of having a family member with chronic pain is unstable emotions. It is okay and predictable to feel different from one moment to the next. When the pain is unpredictable, how can you find steady, stable ground to stand on? Instead you ride the roller coaster of uncertainty, fear, and doubt. Your feelings, unchecked, can actually make matters worse.

Emotional Extremes

Emotional extremes involve the significant imbalances of feeling either too much (overreacting) or too little (underreacting). Emotional imbalance includes not allowing yourself to experience your feelings as they evolve, suppressing or "stuffing" them, or being controlled by or "drowning" in them. Statements that reflect these respective extremes range from "I don't feel anything," "Nothing bothers me," or "I feel numb" to "I can't take it anymore!" "I just want to stop feeling this way!" or "I hate feeling this way!"

Underreacting is an extreme style of emotional responding that involves avoiding both feeling and expressing emotions as much as possible. This can happen unconsciously or as a result of conscious decision making. People with this emotional style rarely, if ever, seem to react with strong feelings. They keep their distance from emotions— they usually don't cry, and seem to treat virtually all situations as if nothing is a big deal. They learned early in life that expressing feelings is something to be avoided, and as a result, dealing with feelings directly—including actually feeling them at all—is unfamiliar, uncomfortable, and unsafe. Such individuals are much more comfortable in the realm of thoughts, thinking, and logic.

Overreacting is an extreme style of emotional responding on the opposite end of the spectrum. People with this style have minimal, if any, distance from the emotions they experience from moment to moment. They act out on their feelings immediately and impulsively and seem to be driven by emotions, with little or no thought or logic. They tend to react to most situations as if they are true crises, living in and constantly creating drama. The urgency and intensity of this drama can have the effect of pulling other people in like a whirlpool and involving them in the scenario. They don't just feel their feelings; they are consumed by them. Many people learned to overreact from growing up in environments where that style is prevalent, where emotions are expressed as soon as they are felt, without any conscious thought about the potential consequences of instantaneous, sometimes reckless venting.

Feelings are neither "good" nor "bad"; they just are. Finding balance with emotions requires moving more to the middle ground of feeling your feelings.

Mary grew up with an alcoholic father. Things were always unpredictable in her house, and as she got older, it got worse. Verbal and emotional abuse prevailed, and toward the end, physical abuse. She left at sixteen and never looked back, except in her memories, which were filled with emotional distress.

Developing Awareness of Emotions

The capacity to identify, feel, and express emotions is essential to a balanced state. Yet many people have great difficulty identifying feelings and expressing them in ways that support emotional balance, especially in challenging situations such as with chronic pain.

There are several levels of awareness involved in cultivating emotional balance. The first level is becoming consciously aware that you are experiencing a feeling. Although you may not know specifically what the feeling is, it is important to simply notice and acknowledge that you have some feeling.

The next step is identifying what the particular feeling is. An important part of identifying your emotions is to put them into words. As an alternative to not knowing what you are feeling or feeling confused, it is helpful to *label* the feeling: "I feel anxious," or "I feel angry," or "I feel depressed." The more specific you can be in identifying your feelings, the more likely you will understand the emotional experience.

*Connecting Emotions to Bodily Sensations*_____

{ *exercise* 8.1 }

Read through the list of feelings in the left column and circle the ones you are experiencing. Next, take a moment to think about them—it may be helpful to close your eyes and turn your focus inward. In the middle column, complete the following sentence about each feeling you are experiencing with the *first thought* that comes to mind: *I feel (emotion) about/because* …. Finally, in the right column, indicate *where* in your body you experience each feeling. For example, anger might be felt as tightness in your shoulders, sadness as an aching in your chest, fear as a knot in your stomach, and joy as warmth in your heart.

Learning how different emotions feel in your body in terms of their location (where you feel them) and sensation (what they feel like) will enable you to identify them more quickly and accurately. Likewise, reading over your sentence completions about each emotion can help you to understand the source of or reason for that feeling.

Emotion	For each emotion, complete the following sentence: "I feel _____ about/ because _____."	Where and how you feel it in your body (e.g., tension in my neck)
Anger		
Resentment		
Fear		
Anxiety		
Grief/Loss		
Depression/Sadness		
Loneliness/Isolation		
Guilt		
Shame/Embarrassment		
Ambivalence/Uncertainty		
Self-pity		
Serenity/Peace		
Love		
Hope		
Gratitude/Appreciation		
Compassion/Empathy		
Other: _____		

Feelings Always Find a Path to Expression

Many families struggling with pain try to deny or stuff their feelings. Our common thought process tells us that if we can just avoid something painful, it won't affect us. However, in the same way that lightning always finds a path to ground, feelings— including painful and uncomfortable ones—always find a path to expression. If we do not address and express them consciously and directly by allowing ourselves to feel them and talk about them, they will come out in indirect forms, often as unhealthy, self-defeating, and/or explosive behavior. When feelings are expressed through behavior, they are typically operating unconsciously and outside our awareness and control.

That being the case, you have a choice in the way you deal with your emotional pain. The choice is to address your feelings in the moment without further damaging yourself or others, or to avoid them and overreact in uncontrolled, dramatic ways. Allowing your painful feelings to be expressed through your behavior only adds more suffering to your life and the lives of others. Emotional balance gives you the capacity to choose which path you will take, instead of letting fear and avoidance make the choice for you.

Emotional Sensitivity

Another variable that can contribute to imbalance is emotional sensitivity. People who are emotionally sensitive feel things more rapidly and more deeply than others and tend to personalize them. Emotionally sensitive people may learn ways to numb themselves from their feelings because so many of their feelings are painful. Feelings of anger, sadness, and depression are not only felt strongly, they are consuming, resulting in intensification of suffering. Negative, uncomfortable emotions can become like a snowball rolling downhill. It gets bigger, gaining strength and speed as it continues. The longer it is allowed to roll without anyone attempting to halt its progress, the harder it is to slow it down or stop it. Chris was edgy and seemed to always bear a short fuse. He hated being this way but couldn't seem to change the way he was feeling.

You may use a range of strategies, including drugs and alcohol, to keep from feeling negative emotions. Drugs and/or alcohol actually increase emotional sensitivity whenever the acute effects of those substances wear off. Use of mood-altering substances can have substantial and adverse affects on your ability to identify, tolerate, and express emotions, creating imbalance in your emotional life.

In pain recovery, you work to restore that balance. The rest of this chapter examines specific emotions that are normal and natural for everyone, but are especially relevant for families dealing with chronic pain.

Fear

Fear is a natural human emotion that can help us to respond effectively to things that threaten us. Walking out into the middle of a busy highway appropriately causes fear. If someone points a gun at you and threatens to shoot you, obviously fear is a rational reaction to the situation. Fear can also be irrational, lacking reason and clarity. Fear becomes problematic when you allow it to debilitate you by keeping you from doing the things you need to do in order to function in the world. Also, it can be troublesome to be consumed by fear about something that *might* happen — anticipating the worst.

Fear feeds on itself; the more fearful you are, the more fearful you become, and the less able you are to function. Some common fears associated with chronic pain are related to life as you knew it being over, the person in pain getting worse or sometimes even getting better, the person in pain falling or being injured when left alone, failed medical procedures or surgeries, addiction, job or career problems, financial problems, relationship problems, or parenting concerns. Many of these fears stem from fear of the unknown and/or fear of change.

Fear can be very difficult to acknowledge to yourself and others. Few people like to admit to or talk about being fearful. In some circles, feeling scared and expressing fear is viewed as weakness, making it even harder to discuss it with others because of the desire to avoid negative perceptions and judgments. Mary was afraid of so many things—losing her job, losing the house, Jim falling, the kids turning out badly. When Jim got hurt, the fear intensified. She hated herself for being a "wuss." Her dad had taught her that being afraid was weakness.

It requires strength and courage to do anything that is uncomfortable or to do things differently from the way you've done them in the past. Therefore, rather than reflecting weakness, admitting to and talking about your fears reflects strength. Keep in mind that courage is not the absence of fear; courage is being aware of your fear and doing what you need to do in spite of it.

{ *exercise* 8.2 }

Learning About Your Fears _____

Identify your greatest fears as they relate to _____'s chronic pain.

_____
_____
_____
_____
_____

Describe specifically what it is about each of the above that creates fear for you.

_____
_____
_____
_____
_____

Describe how living with these fears has affected you.

_____

_____

_____

_____

_____

Anxiety

Anxiety can be thought of as low-level chronic fear. It can be defined as distressing uneasiness, nervousness, or worry felt in response to any situation you *anticipate* to be threatening. It is usually accompanied by self-doubt about your capacity to cope with it. Some of the physical symptoms of anxiety are sweaty palms, increased heart rate, muscle tension, breaking out in cold sweats, inability to sit still, and/or a feeling of being uncomfortable in your own skin. Caring for someone with chronic pain is often the cause of increased anxiety. There are numerous reasons for this, including all of the issues linked to the fears commonly associated with chronic pain. Failure to practice self-care behaviors, such as eating properly, exercising, getting adequate sleep, and relaxation, also contributes to increased anxiety. When you are anxious, remind yourself that your self-care is important and take the time to focus on your personal well-being.

Anxiety can also arise as a result of conflicting feelings or needs, such as between you and family member(s), or within yourself. For example, you may have a strong need for physical affection (e.g., hugs), but because of his or her pain, your spouse shies away from that. Also, if your need for affection has been repeatedly rebuffed for this reason, you may come to feel anxious or fearful of expressing your needs. Conflicting internal feelings can take the form of, for example, finding yourself feeling resentful that your family member does not want to do something (e.g., go out for dinner) because of increased pain, while at the same time thinking you should be more understanding and accommodating. Instead of expressing the feeling you do not think you should feel (e.g., anger, resentment), you may simply feel anxious, nervous, "bad," or trapped and not know why. Again, you may learn to not express your *true* feelings to avoid feeling this anxiety.

Chris never used to worry so much before Amy got sick. He would have trouble sleeping some nights, but now it was three times a week. He felt like he should get some "worry beads," but he wasn't sure where to find them.

An effective way to decrease anxiety is by learning and practicing relaxation and self-calming skills such as meditation, intentional deep breathing, progressive muscle relaxation, guided imagery, self-hypnosis, and even quiet down time. A holistic approach will be most effective in helping you develop healthy habits to continue practicing in order to establish emotional balance. Balanced individuals experience manageable levels of appropriate anxiety. However, if your anxiety is because of conflicting feelings as noted above, you may need to consult with a counselor in order to identify and effectively work through those conflicts.

Some things you can do to decrease anxiety are:

- Reduce/limit caffeine consumption (definitely none after 4:00 p.m.).

- Pay attention to nutrition/limit sugar intake.

- Focus on the present/work on staying in the moment.

- Learn to meditate and practice diligently.

- Read recovery-related materials.

- Exercise as regularly as possible.

- Develop trust in the process of recovery to the best of your ability.

- Pay attention to spirituality—faith in something greater than yourself.

- Practice yoga.

- Practice Chi Kung.

- Explore reiki.

{ *exercise* 8.3 }

Taming Anxiety _____

Identify the issues that bring up the most anxiety for you.

_____
_____
_____
_____
_____

Describe how worrying about these issues is helpful to you.

_____
_____
_____
_____
_____

How much time did you spend last week worrying about things that never happened?

_____

_____

_____

Identify at least three things from the list of suggestions above that you can begin to
practice in order to reduce your anxiety.

_____

_____

_____

_____

_____

Depression, Sadness, Grief, and Loss

Having a family member in chronic pain results in multiple losses—the loss of
the relationship as it once was, loss of shared social and recreational activities,
loss of financial security, loss of hopes and dreams being fulfilled, to name a few.
These losses characteristically lead to feelings of hopelessness, helplessness, and
worthlessness. Not acknowledging or expressing the emotions that arise from these
losses can lead to being stuck in a perpetual, unresolved grief process.

The truth for Mary was that things weren't the way they had been. Jim was unable to
work, and she had to carry the family. She missed their closeness. She missed sexual
intimacy. She was sad about it and continually wished things were different.

The feeling states of sadness, grief, and loss are closely related to one another and
often fall underneath the umbrella of depression. Sadness refers to a feeling of
unhappiness, while grief consists of distress related to the process of mourning a
loss of some sort. Depression can be a feeling but is also a mood—a more enduring
emotional condition that exists on a continuum. Depression is sometimes described
as anger turned inward against oneself. Studies show that an estimated 50 percent
of caregivers are clinically depressed. The most severe form of depression is a
diagnosable disorder marked by a variety of symptoms that can include:

- Sadness.

- Difficulty sleeping or sleeping too much.

- Increased or decreased appetite.

- Weight loss or gain.

- Loss of interest and enthusiasm.

- Feelings of helplessness, hopelessness, and/or worthlessness.

- Decreased self-esteem.

- Fatigue or loss of energy.

- Poor concentration or indecision.

- Suicidal thoughts, thoughts of death, or suicide attempts.

Grief is a natural state attached to loss. The more emotionally important the loss, the greater the grief associated with it. Healing from grief involves mourning the loss and eventually accepting it. Mourning is a process of saying good-bye to and letting go of what you have lost. Acceptance of a significant loss does not mean that there is no longer any distress related to it. Losses that are fully accepted can still be painful, but they no longer create serious emotional imbalances that hinder health and healing. Much like a physical injury that has healed, there may always be a scar. Mourning and healing from grief is a process of regaining balance that takes time (months to years, generally) and is different for each individual. This healing process requires allowing yourself to fully feel all the uncomfortable, painful emotions that are part and parcel of saying good-bye to and letting go of people and things that were important in your life, including, but not limited to, sadness, anger, and depression.

Mood-altering substances actually cause depression, though they seem to relieve it (only temporarily).

{ *exercise* 8.4 }

*Depression and Grief*_____

Identify any symptoms of depression you have experienced.

_____

_____

_____

_____

Describe two things you can do to help you through these symptoms of depression.

_____

_____

_____

_____

Identify your most significant losses, including losses due to chronic pain, and describe how you grieved each one.

_____

_____

_____

_____

_____

_____

_____

_____

Describe your understanding of what you need to do in order to more fully grieve and accept these losses and to heal and regain balance.

_____

_____

_____

_____

_____

_____

Loneliness and Isolation

Loneliness and the tendency to isolate oneself from other people are closely connected to depression, sadness, grief, and loss; however, this is such a fundamental issue for families struggling with chronic pain that we are addressing it separately. Loneliness is defined as a state of sadness specifically because of the emotional experience of being disconnected from others, of feeling and/or being, in reality, all alone. For the person with pain, this feeling may come from a sense of being alone with his or her pain or alone with the disease of addiction and believing that no one understands or can understand his or her situation. For someone in a relationship with the person with pain, this may come from social isolation or may be because of the sense of emotional disconnection because the pain sufferer is preoccupied, distant, and medicated. This experience can be so consuming that some have described it as feeling completely alone even in a crowd of people. Sometimes, the negativity you feel is so severe that even those close to you may withdraw and keep their distance.

Chris was angry at friends for not coming around, but the truth was that he preferred it that way. No one got to see how bad Amy had gotten, and he didn't have to risk their disapproval. "Let them all go to hell," he said in frustration, and his sense of loneliness deepened.

Family members are often increasingly socially isolated because they become so consumed with caring for the person in pain. They may become restricted to the house for fear that if they leave, the person in pain will need them, or may injure themselves or put the house or someone else at risk while medicated. They may limit visitors, not knowing when the person in pain might be overmedicated, and not wanting to answer visitors' questions.

Ongoing loneliness and isolation is a major source of emotional imbalance. Humans need connection to others, and cannot achieve emotional balance without supportive relationships.

{ *exercise* 8.5 }

Combating Isolation _____

Describe the ways you isolate from others.

_____
_____
_____
_____
_____

List the people you feel most closely connected to.

_____
_____
_____
_____
_____

Describe specific actions you can take to better connect with others, including both accepting and offering help.

_____
_____
_____
_____
_____

Anger

Anger is an emotional response to things that don't go the way we want them to. Anger results from the experience of feeling "wronged" in some way. Depending on the situation, anger is a healthy and appropriate emotional reaction. Problems with anger usually occur in how this powerful feeling is expressed. Anger can be expressed along a broad spectrum, from suppressing it (not expressing it outwardly) or keeping it inside to the point where you may not even be aware that you are angry, to exploding, such as with screaming, verbal abuse, or even physical violence. Anger and the resentments it can fuel can cause significant stress and high blood pressure, along with increased muscle tension and increased pain.

Families in pain often direct their anger at each other or at other family and friends, for not understanding, not being supportive enough, or simply because they are in the wrong place at the wrong time. Anger might also be directed at yourself because you are unable to take away the pain or handle everything on your own. It is not uncommon to feel angry or resentful toward the person with pain for not trying hard enough, or for his or her behavior when overmedicated. It is also common to be angry with the health care system, specifically the doctors who were unable to help your family member or who prescribed the medications that he or she became dependent on, or the insurance company that won't pay for his or her next procedure or for disability. You may direct your anger at something or someone when you're really angry at something else. For example, you are angry because _____ is hurting, but you shout at your kids or kick the dog. This is referred to as displaced anger. Frequently, the more anger you have, the more out of emotional balance you are.

In most circumstances, anger is really a secondary emotion. It often forms immediately and automatically (this happens unconsciously, so there may be no awareness of it) in response to a situation that brings up feelings of hurt, fear, and/or inadequacy. Hurt and fear are the primary emotions that anger covers up. When most people experience these primary emotions, they feel vulnerable and their energy and attention are focused internally. This inward focus on one's own vulnerabilities is extremely uncomfortable, especially for individuals who are used to focusing on other people and things outside themselves. Anger serves several defensive purposes. It works as a shield that deflects uncomfortable primary emotions so they can be avoided or kept at a distance. Anger provides a sense of power and control, and directs focus outward to identifiable, external scapegoats. It is almost always easier and more comfortable to focus on the actions of others than it is to focus on yourself.

What can you do about anger? First and foremost, awareness that you are angry is necessary in order to make a conscious decision as to what to do about it. It is helpful to ascertain what you are really angry about—the true reason that you are angry. Knowing the source of the anger and looking beneath the apparent reason ("He's just a jerk") to a deeper level ("My feelings were hurt because he _____") is valuable in examining your emotional reaction. The next steps in dealing with anger are identifying your wants and needs related to what's happening; selecting the solutions that are the best fit from the available options; and then taking action to implement those solutions. This solution-oriented process provides a direct route to finding balance.

{ *exercise* 8.6 }

Evaluating Anger _____

Describe the two most recent instances when you were angry.

_____

_____

_____

_____

_____

Now try to identify the underlying emotions in these situations that your anger may have been keeping under cover, such as hurt, fear, or inadequacy.

_____

_____

_____

_____

_____

Be aware that you almost always play a part in the problems you experience. Identify how you may have contributed to the situation(s) that you were angry about.

_____

_____

_____

_____

_____

Resentments

Resentments are related to anger in that they are negative feelings or ill will directed at someone or something experienced as wrong, unjust, insulting, or disrespectful. Anger is about the present, whereas resentments relate to the past. It is a reexperiencing of past events and the old feelings of anger connected to them. Resentments are created when we get angry at a person, institution, or situation, and hold onto that anger.

People can hold onto resentments for many years, refusing to let go, forgive, or forget, carrying their resentments wherever they go. Like an extra suitcase, they are baggage that weighs them down and requires attention and energy. Over time the person, place, thing, or event that caused the original anger and led to resentment may be forgotten, while the resentment remains like smoldering embers that are left after the flames of a fire have died down. The fire no longer rages, but the embers remain hot and capable of causing more fires in the future unless they are extinguished. As long as these embers continue to burn, they create negative distractions that take time, attention, and energy away from your recovery. As long as you are focused on the people and situations you are angry at and resentful toward, you are out of balance emotionally.

The continuous mental and emotional reenactment of past events that occurs with resentments reinforces feelings of being victimized. Feeling that you have been "wronged" makes you feel like a victim. This makes recovery more difficult because such perceptions interfere with the ability to take responsibility for your own choices and actions. The stronger the resentment is, the more time you spend thinking about it and being caught up in the anger connected to it. This is a form of mental, emotional, and spiritual bondage. Ultimately, the person holding the resentment is the one who suffers most. After all, you can't change the past. So all you can do is shift your focus away from past resentments and toward being as successful as you can in the here and now.

The following are some techniques you can apply to deal with anger and resentments more effectively and regain emotional balance:

- ❧ Treat other people with fairness and compassion, even when you feel angry at or have resentment toward them. Notice what happens when you change how you act toward them in positive ways. They may change how they act with you.

- ❧ Practice expressing your anger and/or resentments in healthier, recovery-oriented ways: Talk about these feelings with *safe, appropriate* people; talk about them without yelling, screaming, threatening, or acting out; write about them; let go of them physically by working out, taking a run, going for a hike, or playing sports.

- ❧ Resist the urge to be a channel for the anger or resentment of others. The anger and resentment of others can be seductive—it can have an almost magnetic pull. Don't buy into it; resist the urge to join in their misery.

- Accept that the past is the past. Give yourself reminders of this whenever you need to.

- Keep in mind that while anger and resentment are normal, natural emotions, you are always responsible for your actions. No one can "make" you do anything. You choose how you act, and the choice you make is your responsibility. Acting out inappropriately can cause regret and further add to your anger and resentment.

- Stop expecting to be perfect.

{ *exercise* 8.7 }

Letting Go of Resentments _____

List some of your resentments.

_____

_____

_____

_____

_____

Write a few ways to decrease their hold on you.

_____

_____

_____

_____

_____

Shame and Guilt

Guilt is an emotion wherein we feel that we've made a mistake. It is defined as a feeling of having committed some wrong or failed in an obligation. Shame, on the other hand, is an emotion where the feeling is that we *are* a mistake. Shame is defined as a painful feeling of humiliation or distress that may be caused by the conscious awareness of wrong or foolish behavior. Often it is not even attached to a specific behavior, but to how we perceive ourselves internally. These two feelings often exist in partnership for people with chronic pain.

The emotional experience of shame is based on a belief that there's something intrinsically wrong with you as a person. Deep inside you feel fundamentally flawed, and believe that everyone knows it. For many people, it is difficult to escape from the burden of shame that has been internalized as a result of growing up in families whose emotional style was to shower their members with shame through an ongoing torrent of put-downs, insults, and blaming. When you are "shame-based," anything you do that is less than exemplary reinforces the belief that you are defective and have been all along.

Mary had internalized a sense of shame as a little girl when she couldn't make her dad stop drinking or help her mom when she was sad. She believed she should have been able to do something, and her helplessness with Jim caused her shame to intensify.

Guilt is emotional distress or discomfort based on the belief that there is a problem related to your behavior, rather than to you as a person. It is ordinarily related to a specific action or an event. "Authentic" guilt can be healthy and helpful insofar as it's a sign that we've violated our own values or a more universal moral code. It helps keep us honest and self-aware in ways that contribute to emotional balance. In contrast, "false" guilt is a sense of responsibility for things that go wrong for which you are not responsible. It is easy to fall into a pattern of guilt-driven self-blame—for not being able to stop the pain, for not being able to do more, for being angry or resentful, or for feeling trapped or wanting out of the relationship. Feelings of shame and false guilt emerge when you begin to believe the lies that other people have told you about yourself.

Chris felt guilty every time he and Amy fought, which was daily. He felt guilty for his thoughts and feelings about Amy and was unable to get relief except when he took one of Amy's Xanax. But the relief was short-lived, and the guilt returned with a vengeance, fueled by more guilt for taking poor Amy's meds.

The direct connection between thoughts and emotions is clear in patterns of guilt and shame that are enhanced by thinking characterized by shame-based statements, such as:

- I should be more patient with her; it's not her fault that she's in pain.

- I shouldn't expect him to be like he was before the injury.

- I should be kinder and more tolerant.

- I should be more patient; I'm being selfish.

- I shouldn't think about what it would be like to be with someone who's healthy.

Shame-based statements sometimes said or thought by family members include:

- What's wrong with you?

- How could you do this to us?

- I wish we had never met.

*Dealing with Shame and Guilt*_____

Describe your strengths and positive qualities.

_____
_____
_____
_____
_____
_____

Identify any lies that other people have told you about yourself that you can stop believing.

_____
_____
_____
_____
_____
_____

Describe how you can use the information above to achieve better emotional balance.

_____
_____
_____
_____
_____
_____

Self-pity

Self-pity is defined as excessive, self-absorbed unhappiness over one's own troubles. It is the emotional state of feeling sorry for yourself, sometimes in exaggerated ways. Self-pity is often a characteristic of chronic pain and addiction—after all, these troubles are very real. But the fact that self-pity often results from significant problems does not make it any less destructive in terms of its impacts on emotional balance. When you are feeling self-pity, you are almost exclusively focused on what is wrong or not working in your life.

Practicing Gratitude/Focusing on the Positive _____

{ *exercise* 8.9 }

A solution-oriented way to regain balance when you're feeling sorry for yourself is to make a gratitude list. This can help you regain perspective and disrupt excessive focus on the negative.

Identify *all* the things in your life you are grateful for (it is important to be thorough).

_____

_____

_____

_____

_____

_____

TWO WOLVES

A Cherokee elder was teaching his grandchildren about life. He said to them, "A fight is going on inside me . . . it is a terrible fight between two wolves. "One wolf represents fear, anger, envy, sorrow, regret, greed, arrogance, self-pity, guilt, resentment, inferiority, lies, false pride, and superiority. The other stands for joy, peace, love, hope, sharing, serenity, humility, kindness, benevolence, friendship, empathy, generosity, truth, compassion, and faith. "This same fight is going on inside you, and inside every other person, too." They thought about it for a minute, and then one child asked his grandfather, "Which wolf will win?" The old Cherokee simply replied, "The one you feed."

—author unknown

The Native American parable about the two wolves that battle for our hearts, minds, and spirits illustrates the importance of focusing on potential solutions as opposed to wallowing in problems, as well as how the choices we make play a central role in that process. Choosing to have conscious contact with positive feelings can help facilitate emotional balance.

Complete each of the following sentences with the first thing that comes to your mind.

For me, love means _____ .

My greatest source of happiness or joy is _____ .

It really touches my heart when _____ .

I feel most at peace when _____ .

I have the most compassion when _____ .

The person I feel closest to is _____ .

The things I appreciate most are _____ .

To me, faith refers to _____ .

I trust that _____ .

I feel grateful when _____ .

Sometimes you may think that you shouldn't feel the way you do. Feelings are neither good nor bad—they simply *are*. In the midst of intense negative feelings, whether fear, anger, depression, or whatever form they may take, it can feel as though they will last forever, like they will never end. It promotes emotional balance to maintain an awareness that all feelings are temporary, and that they will *always* change!

Emotional balance is achieved when you allow yourself to feel whatever comes up, and learn to accept your feelings without judging them. Because your feelings are a part of you, accepting them as they are is an important part of accepting yourself as you are. This is also known as self-acceptance. Whatever positive changes you want to make in your life, acceptance of how and where you are at the present moment is one of the keys to moving forward. Accepting your feelings also takes less energy than trying to avoid or suppress them, and helps maintain balance by eliminating the need for them to recur over and over. Genuine acceptance of your feelings gives you the opportunity to shift your energy to thoughts and actions that facilitate the learning, growing, and healing that can fuel the continuing progress of your pain recovery.

Our focus here is for you to learn and begin to practice strategies to identify and express emotions in ways that promote balance, to deal with distressing and uncomfortable feelings in healthier ways, and to strengthen positive feelings. For example, by setting obtainable goals, you can shift your attention toward gratitude, increased hopefulness, potential solutions, and taking action. Remember, your feelings can't hurt you, but reacting inappropriately to them can.

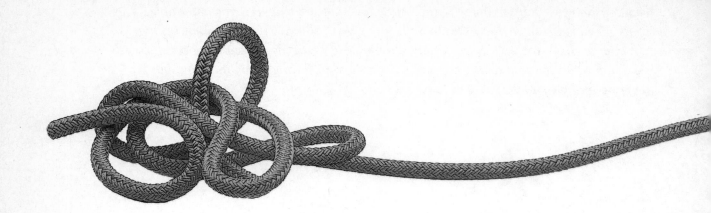

9

Spiritual Balance

In the time since Jim was injured, Mary found herself not wanting to go to church, and did not push going if he said he was in too much pain or the kids wanted to sleep in. She figured, "Why fight it?" Having been fairly regular attendees at Sunday services, more recently they had only been to church on Christmas and Easter. Judy, Mary's good friend at their church, started calling, asking if things were okay and wondering why they weren't coming. Mary just made excuses, citing how much pain Jim was in. But inside Mary knew the real reason they weren't going to church anymore — she was angry at God. Ever since she was a little girl, she had heard her parents and the preacher say that God helps those who help themselves, He only gives you what you can handle, that there is a reason for everything that happens, and that there could be blessings in disguise. She also grew up feeling in her heart that God was kind and good. Now all of these things were questions in her mind. "How could a God who is kind do something like this to us? What possible reason, much less blessing, could there be for Jim's injury and chronic pain?" Mary found herself feeling more and more distant from the strong spiritual connection she had once had in her heart. That once strong connection in the core of her being had been badly shaken, as she no longer saw any point in praying to a God who seemed to give them nothing but suffering in return for their devotion. But she also remembered how at one time the strength of her and Jim's faith had helped them through some other difficult times in their lives. She knew that to survive this journey through chronic pain, she and Jim needed to rediscover their spiritual connection — but how?

In this chapter we will explore some of your basic spiritual beliefs and assist you in understanding the connection between spirituality and your experience of having a family member with chronic pain. What exactly is spirituality? To start, let's consider spirituality as higher emotional functioning. By higher emotional functioning we mean concepts such as faith, hope, trust, belief, unconditional love, and a purposeful life.

- Spirituality can be thought of as the area of life concerned with matters of the spirit, beyond oneself, though not necessarily in the religious sense.

- Spirituality includes a sense of connection to something greater than yourself, which may or may not include an emotional experience of religious awe and reverence.

- Spirituality includes a sense of connection to others, including emotional intimacy, and connection to the world around you—a feeling of belonging to a greater whole.

When we talk about spirituality, it is important to note that we do not mean religion. However, spirituality does not preclude religion. For some, spirituality is closely connected to organized religion and a belief in God. For others, spirituality has absolutely nothing to do with organized religion and/or a belief in God. You can be an atheist and still live a spiritual life. You do not have to believe in a God to live a principle-centered life and believe in the inherent value of yourself and of humankind. The process of recovery allows you the freedom to choose what form your spirituality will take based on the right fit for you.

What Does Spirituality Have to Do with _____'s Pain or Addiction?

Having a family member with chronic pain, especially when addiction is also present, generally results in a lack of hope, faith, and trust. You can become so beaten down by the weight of the pain problem that your worldview becomes pessimistic, the majority of your thoughts center on various forms of doom and gloom, and your relationship to others and the world is increasingly negative.

Chris had never been religious, but believed that someone was watching over him. Recently he had begun to doubt that—how else could he and Amy have ended up the way they were?

Faith, hope, and trust are fundamental components of the pain recovery process. Spirituality helps us reconnect with that which is greater than ourselves and our higher purpose. Spirituality broadens our horizons by lifting us out of a narrow, self-centered focus and helps us find meaning in our difficulties. If you think of pain or addiction as an affliction or a curse; if you think of yourself as a victim; if your frame of mind is one of self-pity, your capacity to experience relief from these burdens and to feel balanced and content will be greatly diminished.

Twelve-step fellowships have demonstrated, over many decades with millions of people, that the concept of coming to believe in a power greater than oneself is an essential part of the process of recovery. This does not mean that you need to "believe" right now, but only that it will be helpful for you do the footwork and see what happens and what beliefs may come out of it. Spiritual beliefs are personal and individual, but we recommend you come to believe in a power greater than yourself that is loving, caring, and nonjudgmental, and only wants what is best for you.

Extremes of Spirituality

Most people would probably acknowledge that too little spirituality could be problematic, but is there such a thing as too much spirituality? In our view, yes—any extreme in one point of balance will result in overall imbalance and interfere with the recovery process.

One spiritual extreme is the rigid, insistent belief that there is nothing greater than the self, no purpose to existence or the universe, and certainly no God. This extreme frequently includes the perception that humankind is inherently "bad" and that people will always attempt to take advantage of you or get over on you if you don't keep your defenses up at all times. This extreme leads to fear, hopelessness, pessimism, distrust, and a sense that life has little or no meaning. Belief in nothing and/or no one beyond oneself swings the pendulum toward cynicism. It also tends to produce resentment toward those who are spiritual. From this perspective, those with spirituality are judged to be weak and dependent: Religion is viewed as the opiate for the masses, and faith is equated with ignorance.

Another extreme is maintaining rigid, inflexible, "set-in-stone" beliefs that you have convinced yourself represent the absolute and only "truth." Most often, this attitude fuels a closed-mindedness that prohibits any actual examination of such beliefs and precludes openness to any other possibilities. This attitude is likely to occur when your concept of spirituality is based solely on religious dogma—positions concerning faith or morality formally stated and authoritatively proclaimed by a specific church or religion, without personal examination. At this end of the spectrum, all other beliefs, forms of spirituality, or conceptions of God typically have to be rejected as false or inferior since your belief is the one true way. In other words, because your belief system must be "right," all others have to be "wrong." This extreme position often breeds the intolerance for all other spiritual perspectives that goes hand-in-hand with religious zealotry. Intolerance is based on the inability to accept that there are alternative forms of spirituality with which your spirituality can peacefully coexist.

Another spiritual extreme is the belief that "God" will take care of everything, and you use this as a reason (or an excuse) *not* to take appropriate responsibility for making decisions and taking actions. When spirituality is seen as a cure-all for life's challenges, it can be used as a rationalization to avoid what you need to do in response to the circumstances life sets before you.

Spiritual Beliefs _____

Describe what spirituality means to you.

_____

_____

_____

_____

_____

Do you believe in God? If so, what is your concept of God? If not, why not?

_____

_____

_____

Has _____'s chronic pain and/or dependence on pain medication affected this belief? If so, how?

_____

_____

_____

To what extent are you angry or resentful regarding religion and/or God?

_____

_____

_____

Describe in as much detail as possible the picture in your mind of who you are and where you are headed in life.

_____

_____

_____

_____

_____

_____

Many Paths

Feeling confused or ambivalent about spirituality is understandable. The most important aspect of developing spirituality is being honest about your feelings, where you are in your life, and what your beliefs are, along with how these beliefs manifest in your perspective, attitude, and behavior. Your challenge here is to be open to the possibility that growing a relationship with a power greater than yourself is a dynamic key to learning how to cope with life in ways that are balanced, healthy, and helpful.

There is no one path on a spiritual journey. In order to find the path that is right for you, you may travel many roads to get to where you need to go. On those roads will be many guides that will help you along the way. There is little to figure out or understand. There is no helpful purpose to be served in trying to find the answers; spirituality is not so much about answers as it is about learning how to appreciate the journey itself. The essence of spirituality is that it's an ongoing quest for meaning and fulfillment.

The parable of the two wolves also applies to your search for spirituality. Isolation, resentments, fear, and anxiety have all fed your imbalance. Here are some things you can do to feed your spirituality and move toward balance:

- Write about your thoughts, feelings, decisions, and experiences daily.

- Read materials that will help you on your path, present you with new information, and open new doors.

- Develop a mutual support system and attend support meetings regularly.

- Take care of yourself physically by staying active, eating properly, and getting adequate rest and relaxation.

- Pray.

- Meditate.

- Share with others.

- Find ways to be of service, to help others.

- Stay present-centered in this moment; live just for today.

- Clear out old resentments and unresolved feelings so you can release these burdens.

- Laugh.

- Be grateful for what you have.

- Accept your situation and cherish the opportunities it provides you to grow and change.

- Make progress toward balancing the four points daily in order to change your experience.

There are no drawbacks to seeking a spiritual experience. You have nothing to lose and everything to gain. All that is required is to be open-minded and willing. On your journey, others may attempt to force their beliefs on you, but you are free to choose what you believe and not believe. Try not to judge your experience or others' experience; just keep moving forward in your journey and notice what happens. There is more joy to be found in the journey than in any particular destination.

Lack of Meaning in Life

Often the majority of meaning we ascribe to our lives relates to what we *do* and what we *have*. In other words, we tend to base the meaning in our lives on our careers and possessions. We commonly spend less time thinking about who we are on the inside and how that gives meaning and purpose to our lives. Material things can never fill internal voids. They may distract attention from internal emptiness or fill some of it temporarily, but such holes can only be filled from the inside. When we neglect who we are in favor of attending to what we do or what we have, our focus will always be outside ourselves and we will miss the meaning of life because that meaning and purpose come from within.

Mary's focus on Jim for the last seven years made her question who she really was. She was a wife, mother, and now breadwinner, nursemaid, and codependent. She felt a real loss of her sense of self and asked herself repeatedly, "Why am I here?"

{ *exercise* 9.2 }

Life Meaning _____

List three things you have (possessions) that contribute to your sense of who you are.

_____
_____
_____
_____

Describe what makes these material things so important to your sense of self.

_____
_____
_____
_____
_____

List three things you do (titles, roles, career) that contribute to who you are.

_____

_____

_____

_____

Describe what makes these things so important to your sense of self.

_____

_____

_____

_____

_____

List five qualities that you consider positive and five qualities that you consider negative that contribute to who you are on the inside.

POSITIVE

_____

_____

_____

_____

_____

NEGATIVE

_____

_____

_____

_____

_____

Describe a minimum of three changes you can start to make to better balance your sense of self from the inside out.

_____

_____

_____

_____

_____

Intuition

An underrecognized facet of spirituality is intuition. Intuition refers to your inner voice that is always there. Being intuitive is similar to common sense, but with differences. Intuition means listening to your inner voice—not the voice in your head, but the voice deep in your heart that tells you if you are doing the right thing. It's usually a quiet voice that requires practice to hear. How many times have you said, "I had a feeling I shouldn't have done that," or "I should have followed my gut feelings"? Some of the variables that make hearing that voice more difficult are fear, anger, resentment, depression, and poor self-care. By practicing pain recovery, you will intuitively make better choices based on what your inner self knows to be healthy for you. By practicing intuitiveness, you take responsibility for your spirituality without just relying on others to tell you what spirituality is or should look like.

Staying in the Moment/Living One Day at a Time

A number of approaches to spirituality emphasize the value of staying in the moment—that is, being present-centered in this moment, right here and right now, as opposed to focusing on what has already happened in the past or could potentially happen in the future. This also extends to the concept of living one day at a time. After all, you can neither change the past nor predict or control the future. The only aspect of time and experience that you have influence in is this moment and today.

There are many ways in which staying in the moment promotes health, healing, and balance. In being present-centered and living just for today, you make yourself genuinely physically, mentally, emotionally, and spiritually available. Focusing on the past or on the future is an exercise in frustration and futility. Helpful techniques to stay in the moment and live just for today include concentrating on and deepening your breathing by paying attention to inhaling and exhaling; focusing on five to ten things in the immediate environment, i.e., the room around you—walls, furniture, ceiling, etc.; and meditation and prayer.

Meditation and Prayer

Meditation is one of the essential components of living a spiritual life. Meditation quiets the chatter in our heads and allows us to gain perspective. The Eleventh Step in twelve-step fellowships talks about prayer and meditation in terms of using these practices as bridges to build a relationship with a power of one's own understanding that is greater than oneself. In this context, prayer is often thought of as a way to *talk to* one's source of spirituality, while meditation is a way to *listen to* that source of spirituality.

One form of meditation is based on mindfulness—that is, enhancing your conscious awareness of your internal experience. Sitting in a comfortable position with your eyes closed, let yourself relax and take note of body sensations, thoughts, and feelings. Notice them without judgment. Let your mind settle into the rhythm of your breathing. If your mind wanders (and it will), gently redirect your attention back to your breathing. Through meditation practice it is possible to face physical pain as well as uncomfortable and painful thoughts and feelings, and to learn simply to accept the pain or anger or sadness and let it pass without obsessing on it or trying to change it. We strongly encourage you to find a meditative discipline that works for you.

Chris regained a little balance when he started meditating. The silence and breath-focus helped relieve his anxiety. For the first time in months, after a yoga class, he felt relief—if only for a moment.

Spiritual Principles

By acting in ways that are consistent with becoming aware of the wishes, feelings, and needs of others, and taking the needs of others into consideration when you make a conscious decision about how you want to act, you will experience greater balance spiritually and overall.

A solution-oriented strategy is to begin to develop a habit of thinking and acting consistent with the Serenity Prayer's guidance to "accept the things I cannot change," where you can accept _____'s chronic pain as a part of your life and counteract it with the spiritual principle of surrender. Remember, paradoxically, surrendering to the things you cannot control or change is necessary to begin to reestablish the ability to choose how you want to act and what kind of life you want to have. One of the most important skills necessary to pain recovery is learning how to cope effectively with the often small but irritating normal and natural frustrations of life.

Developing your spirituality can require ongoing practice of applying such principles as patience, tolerance, acceptance, and humility. Patience is waiting without worrying and enduring without complaint. Tolerance is a spiritual principle that facilitates peaceful coexistence with physical pain and other feelings that are uncomfortable and/or painful, as well as with those people who may annoy, irritate, or otherwise upset you. Acceptance is about being okay with situations and people as they are, rather than focusing on how you want them to be or believe they should be. Humility is not thinking less of oneself, but thinking of oneself less.

The more that you can remain in conscious contact with these spiritual principles, the more balance you will have and the better equipped you will be to accept the full range of experiences that life will present you with.

{ *exercise* 9.3 }

Finding Spiritual Balance _____

Take a moment to list any extremes you are experiencing spiritually.

_____

_____

_____

_____

Describe what you think is needed for you to be balanced spiritually.

_____

_____

_____

_____

What, if anything, is holding you back from achieving this balance?

_____

_____

_____

_____

Another important part of the maintenance of pain recovery is cultivating an attitude of gratitude for whatever blessings you have. Sometimes you may have to look a little harder to see the blessings in your life, but there are always things to be grateful for, no matter how desperate the situation seems. You can learn, perhaps to your surprise, that it is possible to remain in conscious contact with gratitude in spite of feelings of pain, anger, depression, or fear.

When Mary started a gratitude list that her therapist suggested she compile, she was overwhelmed with the many blessings she had in her life. It helped her shift her focus away from her troubles, and she slipped into a state of calm and peace.

A *Gratitude List* _____

In a journal or notebook or on a separate sheet of paper, make a list of all the things you can be grateful for.

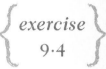

{ *exercise* 9.4 }

The balancing effects of enhanced spirituality may become apparent only gradually over time. It can be weeks or even months after these processes first begin before you realize that your awareness, feelings, and behavior have started to change. When you build a balanced foundation of spirituality that is based on the cornerstones of hope, trust, and faith, you maximize both your internal harmony and the potential for harmony between yourself and others.

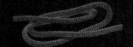

Part III

RECOVER

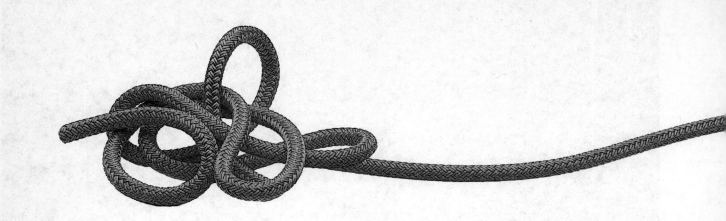

10

Relationships: Finding Mutual Support and Allies

Mary had stopped having visitors over to the house — she didn't want to risk anyone seeing Jim passed out on the couch from too many medications, or in a rage and swearing about how much pain he was in. She had also lost touch with the friends she had made at the gym and in the cooking class she used to attend once a week, since she no longer had time for those things. She felt separated from her family members under her own roof, and separated from everyone outside as well.

Living with someone with chronic pain and/or addiction is guaranteed to result in relationship problems. Your relationships are not only an outward manifestation and an indicator of your overall state of balance; they also affect your state of balance either negatively or positively. While your tendency might be to jump right in and fix your relationships, we caution you that attempting quick fixes will only result in further imbalance. The quickest way to further imbalance in your relationship is to attempt to fix someone else, thinking if he or she were okay, you would be okay. Resist the urge to work on your relationships, and keep the focus on yourself. As you work on your recovery, your relationships will become more balanced. The best way to resolve relationship issues is through slow, incremental changes based on your desire to achieve balance.

Mutual Support and Allies

Human beings are by nature social animals. As such, relationships with other people are of great importance to our overall well-being. In fact, research has demonstrated that social support is an important factor in determining how well someone with a chronic illness is likely to do in the future. Yet, as we've discussed, families who experience chronic pain, with or without addictions, are inclined to isolate themselves socially, effectively cutting themselves off from the balancing and health-enhancing effects of this social support. Research indicates that both loneliness and the pain that contributes to it are significantly lessened by a sense of connection with others, and the distraction offered by interaction with others. This is true whether or not the people who offer the distraction are known and loved by you. Telephone or Internet contact can also provide the double benefit of connection and distraction. Our approach to pain recovery includes seeking balance in this area through connecting with, accepting help from, and offering help to others as a way of life.

{ *exercise* 10.1 }

Connection

Make a list of all activities with other people that you no longer participate in or to a lesser extent since _____ developed chronic pain.

_____

_____

_____

Make a list of all the individuals connected to those activities that you no longer have interaction with or to a lesser extent.

_____

_____

_____

It is important to have people to turn to for support who understand what you are experiencing. Chronic pain is often misunderstood by others. Living in isolation, without the support and encouragement of others who truly understand, will make recovery challenging. Friends, family, and others who are supportive may be helpful, but finding others who have experience with the new path you are on will provide the type of support you need rather than sympathy for your plight.

Amy had been Chris's best friend for the four years they were together. As with many close couples, other friendships became less important. Chris rarely talked to his college buddies and never got close to coworkers, other than an occasional poker game. When Amy got sick, Chris found himself unprepared, unsupported, and feeling alone. The solutions of reaching out became harder to picture, and even harder to execute. He wasn't the type to "dump" his problems on others; he was raised to keep his business private. He felt isolated from everyone and a bit embarrassed to complain to relative strangers. He knew he needed to talk to someone about the progressive deterioration in his life with Amy.

CHRONIC PAIN AND ADDICTION RESOURCES

Many of our clients and their family members have expressed their need for a place they can go to talk about pain and the issues associated with it. Here are some organizations you can contact to find support groups and other resources for family members of people with chronic pain and/or addiction.

Pain in Recovery Support Group (PIRSG): **paininrecovery.org**

Co-Dependents Anonymous (CoDA): **coda.org**

Nar-Anon Family Groups: **nar-anon.org**

Al-Anon: **al-anon.org**

Receiving

Accepting that you cannot deal with the stress of chronic pain or addiction in your family by yourself is essential to help you change old thought patterns and habits. You do not need to be or feel alone as you walk through this process. By building mutual support and allies, you will avail yourself of the personal and spiritual growth that comes from others sharing their experience, strength, and hope with you. Rather than viewing this as taking, look at it as receiving from others. Being able to receive requires admitting there are some things you can't and shouldn't attempt to do on your own. We strongly recommend that you ask for and accept assistance from those who have had a positive experience in areas with which you need help.

When Mary finally called her former best friend Kay, it was like the floodgates opened. When she finally stopped crying and apologizing for being out of touch, Kay insisted on coming over. They sat at the kitchen table for hours—like old times. Jim was feeling okay and came down to sit for a few minutes. When he left, Kay stated, "I don't know who needs more help, Jim or you! But you're my best friend and I'm here to help *you*, so what can I do?" The two childhood friends made lists of the household needs that had overwhelmed Mary for months. Kay put her name next to "pick up Ross at school," "laundry," and "one meal per week." She also committed to calling some other friends to pitch in. Mary felt grateful and caught a glimpse of relief. Kay also suggested Mary look up support groups for families of people with chronic pain, telling Mary, "I can help you with household tasks, but you need to get some help from people who have experienced what you are going through."

Receiving _____

How do you feel about others helping you?

_____
_____
_____
_____

What are your barriers to receiving help from others?

_____
_____
_____
_____
_____

What can you do to overcome them?

_____
_____
_____
_____
_____

Write about your experience with twelve-step fellowships or other group support. Were your experiences positive or negative? Why?

_____
_____
_____
_____
_____

How can you integrate fellowship and supportive people into your recovery?

_____

_____

_____

_____

_____

Giving

After you have received what you need and have achieved some balance in your life, you will be ready to give back to others. Giving completes the circle of balanced relationships. But we must have something in order to give it. Many people think of giving back in terms of time, money, and resources. This is part of giving, but we are also referring to giving back your experience of how you achieved balance in your life. Rather than giving advice, we share solutions and our experience, strength, and hope. We freely give to others what we have received, out of appreciation for what others have given us.

The ability to give back is a gift that recovery provides. When you get out of yourself, it helps you to see your problems in the proper perspective and context. It allows you to focus on things in your life for which you can be grateful.

Giving _____   { *exercise* 10.3 }

Think about what it would be like if, two years from now, you are balanced and content. Write about what you would share with others who are in the same situation as you were. How would you feel about sharing with them? What solutions would you share?

_____

_____

_____

_____

_____

Chris joined a support group for caregivers of people with fibromyalgia, at the suggestion of his therapist. There he was able to talk openly about Amy's fibromyalgia pain. He also started attending a Nar-Anon meeting weekly that a friend recommended, where he was able to address his feelings about addiction, enabling, and codependency. After he broke down and shared in one meeting, people told him how moved they were by his candor and deep emotion. He was helping them be brave and honest—they were helping each other recover.

Relationship Patterns

Relationship patterns are established early in life. Our parents, role models, friends, etc., influence how we view ourselves and others and have an emotional impact throughout our lives. For example, the way you treat others is influenced by the way your parents acted toward each other. If we never examine these patterns we tend to repeat them, no matter how unhealthy they are. You can probably identify several examples in others' lives where you observe repeated dysfunctional behaviors, and you wonder why they keep happening. Identifying your own patterns is a significant step in helping you to choose relationships where you support others and they support you in a mutually beneficial give-and-take.

{ *exercise* 10.4 }

Relationship Patterns

Write about patterns you learned early in life that affect your relationships today.

_____

_____

_____

_____

_____

Write about the changes you'd like to make in these patterns.

_____

_____

_____

_____

_____

Reviewing Your Current Relationships

It is important to take inventory of your current relationships so you can identify those that will help or hinder your quest for balance. We encourage you to assess your current relationships and alter or let go of unhealthy associations and focus on healthy relationships with people who are sincerely interested in your well-being.

Assessing Relationships _____

Make a list of all the significant relationships in your life.

◉ _____   ◉ _____

◉ _____   ◉ _____

◉ _____   ◉ _____

◉ _____   ◉ _____

◉ _____   ◉ _____

◉ _____   ◉ _____

Now review your list and place each relationship into the following categories.

BALANCED AND SUPPORTIVE   **IMBALANCED AND DETRIMENTAL**

◉ _____   ◉ _____

◉ _____   ◉ _____

◉ _____   ◉ _____

◉ _____   ◉ _____

◉ _____   ◉ _____

◉ _____   ◉ _____

If you were able to choose someone to assist you in your pain recovery, what would he or she be like?

_____

_____

_____

_____

_____

Mary found that by getting support from Kay and other friends, she was able to regain a positive sense of herself. Oddly enough, as she became healthier, Jim responded by working harder in his own recovery. It seemed miraculous to her that being with others and sharing made such a difference in the lives of her family. Mandi came around and Ross's grades, and his attitude, improved a lot.

Cultivating and participating in relationships is a crucial part of recovery for families in pain. Playing the caregiver role can leave you isolated and lonely. It is only through sharing your truth by giving and receiving that you can begin to recover. The next chapter will explore actions you can take to enhance your recovery.

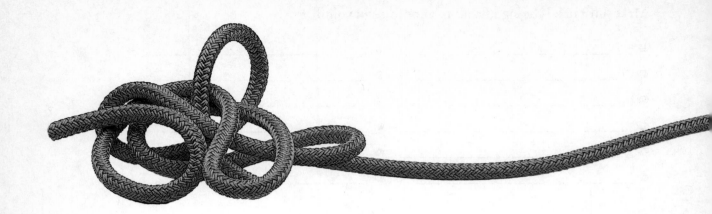

11

Positive Action

Mary felt like a new woman. She was sleeping better, back to the gym, wearing makeup again, and in touch with her circle of friends. She had support in dealing with Jim, and oddly enough, as she became healthier and more comfortable with her new approach to his illness, Jim started getting up more, cut down his medications considerably, and started back with physical therapy. As she got more balanced, Jim responded in positive ways.

When Amy finally got into a pain recovery program, Chris began to feel a call to action. There were things they needed to do together, but just as many each could only do on their own. For example, Chris learned about his tendency to enable Amy's pain and dependence on drugs and the many ways it caused problems for both Amy and their relationship to each other. What still puzzled him, though, was taking care of his own needs. He felt good about getting back into working out again, but still felt guilty about it when Amy was having a bad day with pain and couldn't do much. Sometimes Chris's feelings of guilt nearly stopped him from doing what he knew he needed (and wanted), even though he also knew it would be healthier for him in the long run.

Now that you understand the four points—the essence of who you are—and the kinds of effects they have on your relationships and the world, let's look at how your state of balance will manifest in your life—in other words, your actions and behaviors.

Family recovery maintenance involves continuously monitoring each point and your overall experience, actions, and relationships to stay in balance. Imbalance usually results from not practicing what we've learned in pain recovery. Be careful not to judge yourself for letting up on your recovery—none of us do this perfectly or are always correct and consistent. You simply need to recognize the signs of imbalance and become adept at identifying them as early as possible. Then you can take an action to correct a particular point, get back in balance, and resume recovery. Here, positive action is the key.

Let's look at how each point can become unbalanced and may cause us problems. These are things to watch out for. For each point, we will ask you to create an action plan to return to a balanced state.

Imbalance of Physical Life

Maintaining balance in your physical life entails continuous monitoring, but not judgment, about your state of nutrition, energy, exercise patterns, and ingestion of toxins. It also involves taking care to avoid extremes. If you exercise excessively, you may burn out or injure yourself and stop exercising completely. If your diet is healthy but too strict, you are likely to eventually overindulge and return to unhealthy eating habits. Maintaining physical balance involves monitoring your body as well as emotions associated with your body. Imbalance of the body can manifest as fatigue, aching, nausea, and sleep disturbance.

{ *exercise* 11.1 }

*Creating an Action Plan for Physical Balance*_____
Describe what happens when you don't get enough sleep.

_____
_____
_____
_____
_____

Describe what happens when you eat unhealthy foods.

_____
_____
_____
_____
_____

Describe what happens when you don't exercise regularly.

_____
_____
_____
_____
_____

What are some other physical issues that make you feel imbalanced?

_____

_____

_____

_____

_____

ACTION PLAN

When I can't sleep, I will take the following actions:

_____

_____

_____

_____

_____

When I am not eating right, I will take the following actions:

_____

_____

_____

_____

_____

When I feel run down, I will take the following actions:

_____

_____

_____

_____

_____

When I have other physical problems, I will take the following actions:

_____

_____

_____

_____

Here is a series of physical actions I'm committed to taking on a regular basis:

_____

_____

_____

_____

_____

_____

Imbalance of Thoughts

How you think influences how you feel, which affects your actions. It is difficult if not impossible to have irrational thoughts and not act out with irrational behaviors. If you forget that you are in control of your life and return to feeling like a victim, you may find yourself asking, "Why me?" Freedom from victim-thinking is realizing that "Why not me?" makes much more sense. It can be helpful to remind yourself that you are one of millions who have the same problems or worse.

Be mindful of the messages you are telling yourself. Negative self-talk about the futility of any effort, feeling sorry for yourself, and believing that others really don't understand what you're going through are manifestations of being out of balance. Feeling unique and different will make you less likely to look to others for help or have any interest in helping someone else, leaving you out of balance and in dangerous territory.

When Amy came home from rehab, Chris found himself walking on eggshells. He was sure that relapse was just around the corner. She seemed better than she had been in years, but he felt convinced it wouldn't last. His therapist pointed out his negative thinking and provided positive approaches to deal with his negativity.

Creating an Action Plan for Mental Balance _____

What negative thoughts are you believing or having trouble shaking loose?

_____

_____

_____

_____

_____

How might you challenge those negative thoughts?

_____

_____

_____

_____

_____

What other thoughts come up that get you out of balance (e.g., black-and-white thinking, making things worse than they are, etc.)?

_____

_____

_____

_____

_____

ACTION PLAN

List what actions you need to take when each of the negative thoughts you listed comes up:

_____

_____

_____

_____

_____

Imbalance of Emotions

It is common in life to experience challenging situations that provoke negative emotions. Our responses are difficult, though not impossible, to change. You may experience emotional imbalance in the form of fears (rational and irrational), anger, anxiety, sadness, and frustration. You may also find yourself feeling excitement, happiness, and even elation. These feelings may come up in ways you're not used to dealing with; it is the challenge of dealing with emotions in an appropriate, healthy manner that finding balance will provide.

Having feelings and not being aware of them is another aspect of emotional imbalance. Unless you know what you are feeling, you may fall victim to these feelings and be powerless to control them.

It takes hard work to change these patterns, the kind of work you have done so far. But to sustain the changes, continuous vigilance about your emotional responses to circumstances that arise in your life will be required.

Chris was petrified that Amy would relapse. He loved her so much, but over the years had successfully walled off the loving feelings. Now that she seemed better, he was having difficulty believing he could trust her—that loving her was safe and that she would stay clean. And now that she was back, he found himself getting angry at her for little things. He gradually got in touch with overwhelming anger at her for all she had put him through. He needed to find a healthy outlet for this anger, forgive her, and move on—no easy task!

{ *exercise* 11.3 }

*Creating an Action Plan for Emotional Balance*_____

Emotions may arise when we are not aware or paying attention. Take some quiet time and write about what it's like to:

Feel angry or frustrated with _____.

_____

_____

_____

_____

Feel afraid or uncertain about _____.

_____

_____

_____

_____

Feel lonely or sad about _____.

_____

_____

_____

_____

Feel happy and successful about _____.

_____

_____

_____

_____

ACTION PLAN

What actions you will take when you have negative emotions?

_____

_____

_____

_____

Imbalance of Spirituality

Since spirituality is so individualized, the ways we get out of balance are unique. Some patterns to watch out for include losing a sense of God or higher power and not praying, meditating, or using other spiritual practices. Sometimes neglecting one's spiritual practice can be a sign of anger toward God or a higher power that needs to be dealt with. Becoming self-reliant, isolated, and self-consumed may lead to engaging in unhealthy behaviors. Conversely, becoming overzealous and neglecting family, work, friends, and other activities for spiritual practice is another form of imbalance to watch out for.

Chris's meetings provided an avenue for him to reconnect to his sense of spirituality. People talked about "higher power" in his Nar-Anon meetings, and he became more comfortable allowing God back in his life. This allowed a healing force to enter his life with Amy, and he felt more comfortable than he had in years. They were able to share a common ground of spirituality though they had come from different religious backgrounds.

Creating an Action Plan for Spiritual Balance _____

How have you become removed from your spiritual "comfort zone" in the past?

_____

_____

_____

_____

Describe challenges for which you can allow for a power greater than yourself in your life.

_____

_____

_____

_____

ACTION PLAN

List the actions that bring you closer to your spiritual self and that you will maintain to stay in spiritual balance.

_____

_____

_____

_____

_____

Connecting the Points of Balance

THE RELATIONSHIP BETWEEN THOUGHTS AND EMOTIONS

A common misconception is that emotions or feelings occur in direct response to a sensory event. Such events can be internal, such as our physical state (e.g., a backache), or external to us (e.g., being stuck in traffic). So it may seem that the event causes the resulting emotion. Yet, in response to an event, thoughts actually occur before feelings. It is the way we think about the event, our beliefs about it and how we interpret it, that creates our emotional response. Our emotional response, or the way we feel about an event, then, has great influence over our consequent actions.

This helps explain how different people can experience basically the same event and have completely different feelings in response to it. For example, two women are waiting to be picked up by their husbands after work. They were expecting to be picked up at 5:00 p.m. and it is now 5:20. The automatic thoughts that occur to the first woman go something like: "He's so late. He obviously doesn't care about me enough to get here on time!" In contrast, the thoughts that come up for the second woman are: "He's so late. Traffic must be especially heavy." Based on those different thoughts, and the divergent beliefs about the same situation that those thoughts represent, the emotions each of these women feels are likely to be very different. Place yourself in each position for a moment, thinking each of those different thoughts. What feelings come up for you in response to each set of thoughts?

In response to this same event, there are multiple different thoughts that could occur automatically, including, but not limited to: "He must have forgotten about picking me up"; "I wonder if everything's okay"; "Maybe the kids' practice ran late"; "I hope he didn't get into an accident." Each of these thought responses has different beliefs or interpretations attached to it, and, in turn, each belief or interpretation is likely to generate different feelings in response to the same event.

Connecting Thoughts and Emotions _____ { *exercise* 11.5 }

Describe an event you have experienced where the initial thoughts you had and your beliefs about _____ turned out to be inaccurate.

_____

_____

_____

_____

_____

Identify the feelings that came up for you in response to your thoughts about _____ and this event.

_____

_____

_____

_____

Imagine yourself back in the situation and change your initial thoughts and beliefs so that they match what actually happened. Identify the feelings that come up for you now in response to these changes in your thoughts and beliefs about the event.

_____

_____

_____

_____

Notice how different the feelings that came up for you were after you changed your initial thoughts and beliefs to accurately fit the situation, compared to your first set of feelings.

HOW DOES THIS PROCESS RELATE TO LIVING WITH A PERSON WITH CHRONIC PAIN?

If, in our example, it were you waiting to be picked up after work by your spouse who has a chronic pain condition, and your automatic thoughts and the beliefs related to the event are negative (e.g., "He's so lazy! Can't he even pick me up on time?" or "Maybe he's using drugs again and that's why he's late"), the emotions that result are frustration and/or anger. Frustration and anger lead to conflict or tension between you and your spouse.

This increased tension can result in unspoken suspicions, resentments, and concerns on your part, as well as increased pain for the chronic pain sufferer. There is a correlation between negative thinking and beliefs and the level of pain a person experiences—the more negative the thoughts and beliefs, the greater the pain sensations. So there can be discomfort or pain triggered in both of you, as well as conflict triggered within your relationship to each other. It can quickly become a vicious cycle. The longer such a cycle continues, the more out of balance you may become.

The progression is essentially as follows:

Event (overshadowed by chronic pain)

Negative thoughts/self-talk/beliefs

Suffering/anger/depression

Tension and stress

Conflict between you and increased pain for chronic pain sufferer

Increased negative thoughts/self-talk/beliefs

Greater suffering

The process of pain recovery includes dramatically changing this negative progression through regaining balance in thinking.

Reestablishing balance counteracts this negative progression thus:

Decreasing negative thinking/self-talk

Decreased feelings of frustration, anger, depression, hopelessness, and helplessness

Lower stress and tension

Less conflict, or conflict resolution and less pain

From Thoughts to Actions

We all move through a process from sensing and thinking to actions, and this process usually occurs at time-warp speed. Generally speaking, it does not feel like a multipart process, though it is. The process is unique for each of us and is affected by many factors, but it is possible to lay out a template or outline for healthy and balanced thinking and decision making. A simplified way to represent this process is captured in the following graphic, courtesy of Johanna Franklin and Rob Hunter, psychologists specializing in addictive disorders:

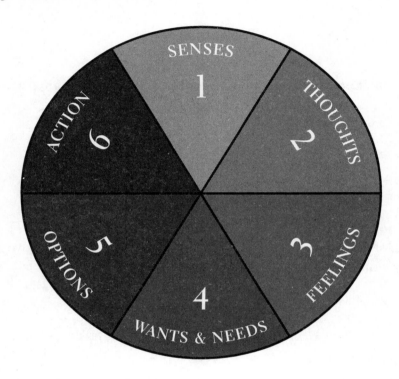

If you picture thought as a six-step sequence, it might look something like the above.

STEP ONE
Sensory perceptions: We perceive events and integrate multiple sensory inputs.

STEP TWO
Thoughts: The integrated sensory experience becomes thought—our brain generates thoughts related to what we sense, and we attach beliefs to the thoughts as to what they mean.

STEP THREE
Feelings: We feel emotions that flow from our thoughts and the beliefs we attach to them.

STEP FOUR

Wants and needs: We determine, based on our feelings, what it is we want and need relative to our specific thought(s). Step four is essentially a business plan in which we figure out what it is we need to happen.

STEP FIVE

Identify and consider options: We examine the options or choices that are open to us to get step four accomplished, and select the best one with which to meet the identified needs.

STEP SIX

Take action: We implement the option/solution we determine to be the best fit for us.

When our thinking is healthy and balanced, we are progressing through these six steps on a fairly continuous basis, though most of us are not consciously aware that we're engaged in this process.

It is common for twists and inaccuracies in thinking to contribute to the train of thought becoming derailed and out of balance. When your family is affected by chronic pain and/or addiction, the above process usually includes only steps one (sensing), two (thinking, typically in strictly automatic, unconscious form), and six (action). Steps three (feeling), four (considering wants and needs), and five (identifying options) are often either short-circuited or completely absent.

In your role as _____'s caregiver, you may have a tendency to avoid spending time on step three because you have become so focused on his or her needs that you no longer consider your own feelings and needs. Skipping or mislabeling the feelings step makes it difficult to establish what it is you're really trying to get done (step four), and if you can't accurately identify your wants and needs, your ability to generate options that meet those needs effectively is seriously impaired. Omitting or shortcutting any steps in this sequence can easily lead to imbalances in how you think.

Anytime Jim would moan in pain, Mary would automatically come running. Her thoughts were always focused on what needed to be done next, crowding out any consideration of how she felt or what she wanted. At first when she began her own recovery process, she found it hard to get back to thinking about how she felt separate from Jim, but with practice she discovered she had many options that she hadn't seen before. To her surprise, she also found that she was a better mate to Jim when she was a more complete and productive person outside the house.

One method we have had success with in the past is to have people visualize the brain as a muscle that has partially atrophied. That is, the "two-three-four-five" muscle group needs to be consciously taken to the mental gym and exercised. Simply getting in the habit of reminding yourself to slow your thinking down a little and make sure that you have properly identified your thoughts and feelings before deciding what needs to be achieved is a helpful skill to practice.

{ *exercise*
11.6 }

Thought-to-Action Process _____

Take this opportunity to put this six-step process into practice. Imagine that an event or situation is being affected by _____'s pain, and you are tempted to suggest medication. Apply the six steps. First, briefly describe the event or situation.

_____

_____

_____

_____

STEP ONE
Describe your sensory perceptions of the event.

_____

_____

_____

STEP TWO
Describe the thoughts that come up for you related to this event.

_____

_____

_____

STEP THREE
Describe your feelings that flow from your thoughts and beliefs related to this event.

_____

_____

_____

STEP FOUR
Identify your wants and needs related to this event.

_____

_____

_____

STEP FIVE

Identify the options that are available to meet your wants and needs related to
this event.

_____

_____

_____

Select the best option available to meet your identified needs.

_____

STEP SIX

Describe the action you will take to implement the option/solution you selected.

_____

_____

_____

Get Into the Solution

Pain recovery is solution-based. It applies the principles of the Twelve Steps in the
context of families suffering from the effects of chronic pain in one of its members.
One of the goals of pain recovery is to help you to stop feeling like a victim of your
family member's chronic pain. Living in pain recovery requires acceptance, hope,
a positive attitude, and action. Once you can accept that you are powerless over
_____'s chronic pain, you can begin your recovery process.

Just by reading up to this point, you have taken a huge step toward pain recovery.
Now it gets more difficult, because the process requires you to do things that you may
not want to do. However, those are often the things that are best for us—for example,
going to a support group or a Nar-Anon meeting when you'd rather not or when your
head tells you, "Not tonight. I had a long day and just want to take two Tylenol and go
to bed. I don't feel like 'feeling' the emotions that come up when I'm at a meeting."
Getting into the solution is learning to develop a relationship with a power greater
than yourself, and being open-minded enough to consider this concept. It's opening
up to a counselor or therapist when you don't feel like talking. It's receiving the life-
changing gifts of recovery and then giving back what was so freely given to you.

The path of healing is narrow, since changing your life takes effort and willingness, but immensely rewarding. In order to experience growth that produces change, you *must* look at yourself honestly and learn how to use the tools that will allow you to heal.

This chapter has defined the last piece of the puzzle of your pain recovery. You have seen examples of imbalance and identified actions to correct the imbalances in each of the four points. We looked, in-depth, at the crucial interaction between thoughts and emotions and described how short-circuiting the process has led to imbalanced actions and behaviors. Now it's time to sum up, consolidate your learning, and create a pain recovery plan that you and your family will be able to follow for the rest of your lives together.

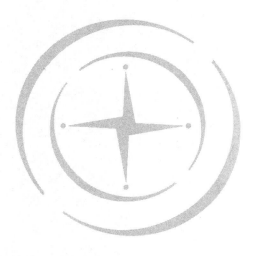

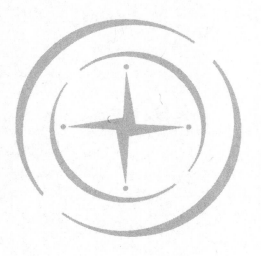

Continuing the Journey
A Long-Term Pain Recovery Plan

Having a plan of continuing action after completing this book is essential to ensuring an ongoing healthy lifestyle in pain recovery. These next steps that you take will set the tone for your continued recovery, as well as solidify everything you have learned in the previous chapters. Please complete the following recovery plan to the best of your ability. Do not hesitate to ask others who are supportive of your efforts to assist in completing this plan.

Go back in this book and review the exercises you have completed. In each chapter, highlight in yellow the key things you have learned from each chapter. List these items; try to consolidate them into one phrase each.

Chapter One: Understanding Chronic Pain

1.

2.

3.

4.

5.

Chapter Two: How Families React to Chronic Pain

1.

2.

3.

4.

5.

Chapter Three: Chronic Pain and Addiction: Double Trouble

1.

2.

3.

4.

5.

Chapter Four: Is It Addiction?

1.

2.

3.

4.

5.

Chapter Five: Pain Recovery: Finding Balance

1.

2.

3.

4.

5.

Chapter Six: Physical Balance

1.

2.

3.

4.

5.

Chapter Seven: Mental Balance

1.

2.

3.

4.

5.

Chapter Eight: Emotional Balance

1.

2.

3.

4

5.

Chapter Nine: Spiritual Balance

1.

2.

3.

4.

5.

Chapter Ten: Relationships: Finding Mutual Support and Allies

1.

2.

3.

4.

5.

Chapter Eleven: Positive Action

1.

2.

3.

4.

5.

Now prioritize these as accurately as you can—in other words, in each chapter rank them from one to five in order of importance, with one being the highest importance.

List the top item from each chapter and rank those eleven items in order of importance from one to eleven.

1.

2.

3.

4.

5.

6.

7.

8

9.

10.

11.

As you can see, you have a good idea of the important things you have learned from this book.

Now list concerns—these are issues that might be called "triggers." Include any issues that come to mind as potential trouble areas that might result in wanting to return to dysfunctional behavior patterns. Return to the previous chapters and circle problem areas in green. List at least ten here.

1.

2.

3.

4.

5.

6.

7.

8.

9.

10.

One more time, return to the text and extract or think of possible solutions for each of the potential triggers. For example, when I feel afraid I will pray, call someone reliable, read certain pages, and write about them.

1.

2.

3.

4.

5.

6.

7.

8.

9.

10.

List specific steps that you will take to avoid unhealthy thoughts, negative feelings, physical problems, and spiritual disconnection.

1.

2.

3.

5.

6.

7.

8.

9.

10.

BALANCE INVENTORY WORKSHEET

1. Stop and take a deep, slow breath.

2. Notice your state of each point of balance. What's going on in your body, mind, emotions, and spirit? Write your observations in the table below.

Physical	Mental	Emotional	Spiritual

3. Are these observations familiar or new? What can you compare them to?

_____

_____

_____

_____

_____

_____

4. Picture your life with balance in all four points. What does it look like? What feelings does it bring up? In the table below, write about the mental picture you created of your life in balance and the feelings you have about it.

Physical	Mental	Emotional	Spiritual

5. What do you need to do in order to have the life you pictured? Set goals and create an action plan to make adjustments and changes in any areas that are imbalanced.

GOALS

1. _____
_____
_____

2. _____
_____
_____

3. _____
_____
_____

4. _____
_____
_____

5. _____
_____
_____

ACTION PLAN

_____
_____
_____
_____
_____

6. Contact someone from your support system and discuss what you've written.

Recovery Support

List the twelve-step meetings or other support groups that you are going to attend on a weekly basis.

Day	Time	Location

Appointments and Sessions

Make a list of your appointments and sessions with, for example, a counselor, psychologist, physician, or any other provider who can assist in your recovery plan.

Name	Date and Time	Type of Service

Recovery Reading and Writing Materials

List books, articles, or other materials that you will use to assist in your ongoing recovery.

_____
_____
_____
_____
_____
_____

The success of your pain recovery truly depends on how well you choose to follow this recovery plan and your willingness to do so. Recovery is a lifelong process that does not stop after completing this book; in fact, this is just a beginning.

Remember that balance is a fluid, ever-changing process, so be good to yourself and make gentle, incremental changes when needed. Take this plan and post it someplace where you can look at it each and every day to remind you of the positive things that you need to do on a regular basis to stay balanced.

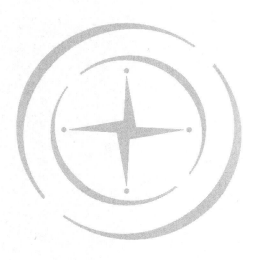

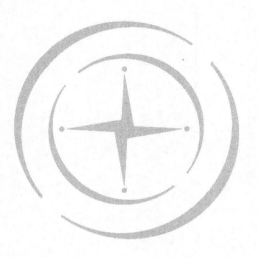

COMPANION PIECES FOR
PAIN RECOVERY FOR FAMILIES

A Day without Pain
Mel Pohl, MD, FASAM with Mike Donahue

In a concise, easy-to-read format, *A Day without Pain* offers a thorough explanation for the mechanisms of pain, opioid use, and addiction, and reviews opioid-free solutions that bring relief from chronic pain.

My Pain Recovery Journal

A specialized journal designed to be compatible with *Pain Recovery* that gives those dealing with chronic pain a separate space for recording thoughts, expressing feelings, and monitoring progress. Also contains writing prompts to promote journaling that enhances the pain recovery process.

Pain Recovery: How to Find Balance and Reduce Suffering from Chronic Pain
Mel Pohl, MD, FASAM; Frank J. Szabo, Jr., LADC; Daniel Shiode, Ph.D.;
Robert Hunter, Ph.D.

Pain recovery is a different approach to pain management and a lifestyle that encompasses a person's mind, body, emotions, and spirit. This method offers a healthy, opioid-free way to live with chronic pain and minimize suffering. The four authors offer the techniques, lessons, and exercises needed to reduce pain without drugs; based on a pain rehabilitation program that has helped change the lives of many.

Meditations for Pain Recovery
Tony Greco

Based on the ideas and discoveries presented in *A Day without Pain* and *Pain Recovery*, *Pain Recovery Meditations* provides 365 entries for those in recovery from chronic pain and co-occurring addiction. Entries address both pain recovery and addiction with an eye to developing the reader's "four points of balance," physical, spiritual, mental, and emotional, with suggested meditations for each day of the year.

To order or find more information on these and other
Central Recovery Press titles, visit CentralRecoveryPress.com

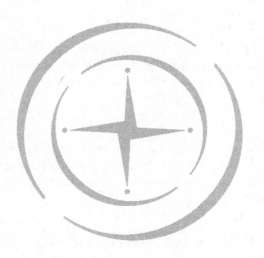

REFERENCES

Chapter One
Understanding Chronic Pain

Farber, PL, J Blustein, E Gordon, and N Neveloff. "Pain: Ethics, Culture, and Informed Consent to Relief." *Journal of Law, Medicine & Ethics* 24, no. 4 (1996): 348–59.

National Center for Health Statistics. "Chart Book on Trends in the Health of Americans with Special Feature on Pain." In *Health, United States, 2006*. Hyattsville: CDC National Center for Health Statistics Press, 2006.

Pohl, M. *A Day without Pain*. Las Vegas: Central Recovery Press, 2008.

Society for Neuroscience. "Brain Briefings: Gender and pain." May 2007. http://web.sfn.org/index.cfm?pagename=brainbriefings_gender_and_pain.

Chapter Two
How Families React to Chronic Pain

Bufalari, L, T Aprile, A Avenanti, F Di Russo, and SM Aglioti. "Empathy for Pain and Touch in the Human Somatosensory Cortex." *Cerebral Cortex* 17, no. 11 (2007): 2553–61.

Flor, H, et al. "Conditioning: Learning that Pain Can Elicit Reward." Society for Neuroscience Annual Meeting (2002).

Jackson, PL, A Meltzoff, and J Decety. "How Do We Perceive the Pain of Others? A Window into the Neural Processes Involved in Empathy." *Neuroimage* 24, no. 3 (2005): 771–79.

Saarela, MV, Y Hlushchuck, AC de C Williams, M Schurmann, E Kalso, and R Hari. "The Compassionate Brain: Humans Detect Intensity of Pain from Another's Face." *Cerebral Cortex* (Oxford) 17, no. 1 (2007): 230–37.

Society for Neuroscience. "Findings on Pain, Including How a Spouse Can Spur the Sense, Provide New Insights." 2002. http://www.sfn.org/index.cfm?pagename=news_11032002a.

Chapter Three
Chronic Pain and Addiction: Double Trouble

Manchikanti, L, K Cash, K Damron, R Manchukonda, V Pampati, and C McManus. "Controlled Substance Abuse and Illicit Drug Use in Chronic Pain Patients: An Evaluation of Multiple Variables." *Pain Physician* 9 (2006): 215–26.

National Institute on Drug Abuse. "Drugs, Brains, and Behavior - The Science of Addiction." National Institute of Health. http://www.nida.nih.gov/scienceofaddiction/index.html.

Chapter Four
Is It Addiction?

National Institute on Drug Abuse. "Addiction Is a Chronic Disease." National Institutes of Health. http://www.drugabuse.gov/about/welcome/aboutdrugabuse/chronicdisease/.

National Institute on Drug Abuse. "Drugs, Brains, and Behavior - The Science of Addiction." National Institutes of Health. http://www.nida.nih.gov/scienceofaddiction/index.html.

Chapter Six
Physical Balance

Barnard, N. *Foods That Fight Pain.* New York: Three Rivers Press, 1999.

Bronfort, G, M Haas, RL Evans, and LM Bouter. "Efficacy of Spinal Manipulation and Mobilization for Low Back Pain and Neck Pain: A Systematic Review and Best Evidence Synthesis." *Spine* 4, no. 3 (2004): 335–56.

Eisenberg, D, R Davis, S Ettner, S Appel, S Wilkey, M Van Rampey, and R Kessler. "Trends in Alternative Medicine Use in the United States, 1990–1997: Results of a Follow-up National Survey." *Journal of the American Medical Association* 280 (1998): 1569–75.

Kabat-Zinn, J. *Full Catastrophe Living: Using the Wisdom of Your Body and Mind to Face Stress, Pain, and Illness.* New York: Bantam Dell Publishing Group, Inc., 1990.

National Center for Complimentary and Alternative Medicine. "Health Topics A–Z." http://nccam.nih.gov/health/atoz.htm.

Tindle, H, R Davis, R Phillips, and D Eisenberg. "Trends in Use of Complementary and Alternative Medicine by US Adults: 1997–2002." *Alternative Therapies in Health and Medicine* 11 (2005): 42–49.

Wolsko, P, D Eisenberg, R Davis, R Kessler, and R Phillips. "Patterns and Perceptions of Care for Treatment of Back and Neck Pain: Results of a National Survey." *Spine* 28 (2003): 292–98.

Chapter Seven
Mental Balance

National Alliance for Caregiving & Evercare. Study of Caregivers in Decline: A Close-up Look at the Health Risks of Caring for a Loved One. Bethesda, MD: National Alliance for Caregiving and Minnetonka, MN: Evercare (2006).

Chapter Eight
Emotional Balance

Zarit, S. Assessment of Family Caregivers: A Research Perspective. In Family Caregiver Alliance (Eds.), Caregiver Assessment: Voices and Views from the Field. Report from a National Consensus Development Conference (2006): 12–37. San Francisco: Family Caregiver Alliance.

Chapter Ten
Relationships: Finding Mutual Support and Allies

The Lewin Group Inc. National Family Caregiver Support Program Resource Guide (2002). Falls Church, VA: The Lewin Group Inc.

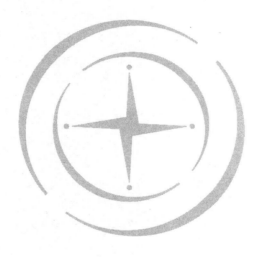

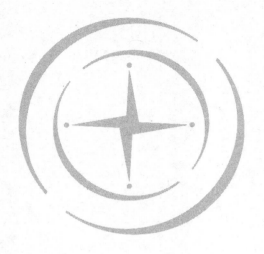

INDEX

Chronic Pain Rehabilitation Program, 56

codependency, 23, 24, 151

Co-Dependents Anonymous (CoDA), 59, 149

complementary and alternative medicine, 84, 89

connection, 148

connections
mind and body, 111

D

denial, 23, 58

depression
caregivers and, 119
symptoms of, 83, 119, 120

distraction, 148

drug dependence, 35, 46

E

emotional sensitivity, 115

emotions
expressing, 114, 119
identifying, 113, 124

empathetic reaction, 26

enabling, 20, 23, 24, 31, 151

exercise, 6, 23, 25, 27, 47, 51, 62, 63, 80, 81, 82, 86, 89, 108, 140, 156

expectations, 106, 107, 108

extremes
emotional, 112
mental, 94, 95
physical, 80
spiritual, 135

F

faith, 134

family
adaptability, 20, 21
cohesion, 20, 21
communication, 20
dynamics, 20
homeostasis, 20
interaction patterns, 20
roles, 18, 20, 22

family system, 18, 20, 21, 31, 61

fear, 4, 8, 15, 30, 49, 56, 87, 115, 116, 117, 122, 123, 124, 129, 130, 135, 137, 140, 143

feelings. *See* emotions

fibromyalgia, 3, 7, 8, 55, 151

four points of balance, XVI, 65, 75, 187

Friel, John and Linda, 24

G

giving, 56, 59, 151, 153

gratitude, 103, 104, 129, 131, 143

grief, 4, 119, 120, 121

guilt, 18, 24, 64, 107, 126, 127, 128, 129, 155

H

hope, 31, 67, 129, 133, 134, 143, 149, 151, 163

humility, 129, 142

hydrotherapy, 11, 87

hyperalgesia, 5, 11, 36, 50

hypnotherapy, 87

I

imbalance

    causes of, 63

    emotional, 64, 112, 160

    mental, 64

    physical, VIII, 63, 80

    spiritual, 64

intuition, 140

isolation, 24, 64, 121, 122, 148

J

journaling, XVII, 187

L

Las Vegas Recovery Center, 56

loneliness, 121

M

massage, 11, 86, 87, 89

medical care, 84

meditation, 65, 86, 117, 140, 141

mindfulness, 141

muscle relaxants, 11

music therapy, 88

mutual support and allies, 147

N

Nar-Anon Family Groups, 59, 149

negative thinking, 95, 158

nonopioid medications, 14

nutrition, 80, 82, 118, 156

O

omega-3 fatty acids, 83

opioid-induced hyperalgesia.
    See hyperalgesia

opioids, 12, 13, 33, 35, 38, 46, 51, 99

    length of use, 11

    withdrawal, 36

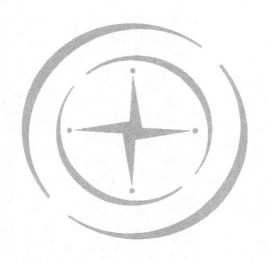